A PARADOX OF VICTORY

A PARADOX OF VICTORY

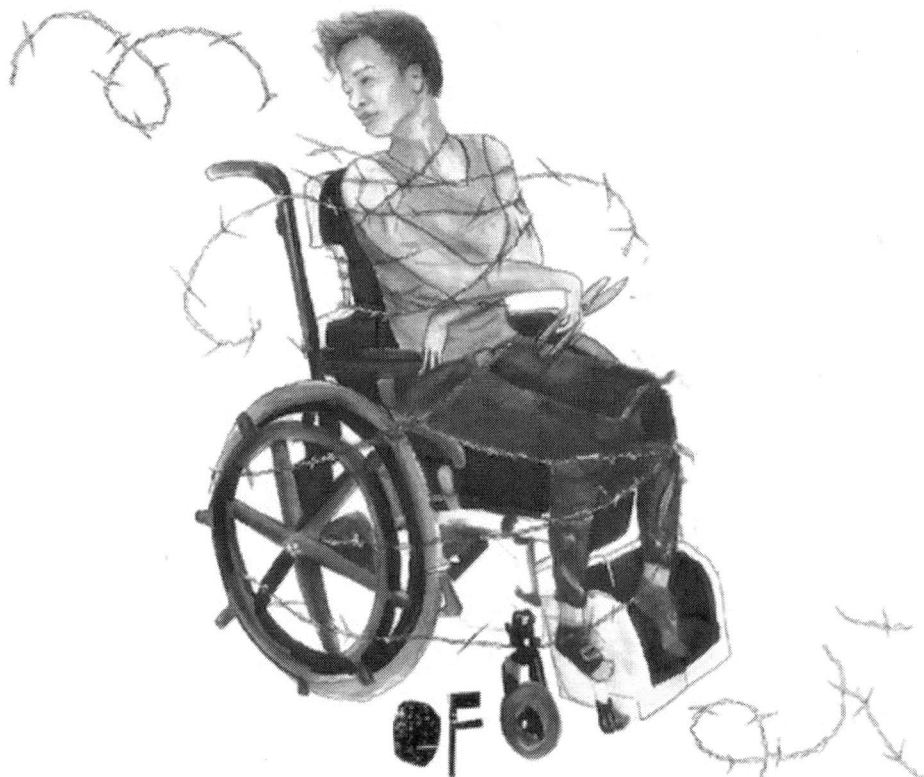

BY NISSI SALAZAR
with Sheri Hunt

A PARADOX OF VICTORY

Printed in the United States of America

First printing, 2018

ISBN-13: 978-1725619913

ISBN-10: 1725619911

Self published by Nissi Salazar

Printed by Kindle Direct Publishing, kdp.amazon.com/en_US

Book cover designed by Benjamin Mayer

Illustrations by Jeanette Dillard, www.jeanettedillard.com

Edited by Susan Macias and Rebecca Siedschlag

10 9 8 7 6 5 4 3 2 1

Acknowledgments...

I couldn't have written this book without the love and support of some very special people:

Momma and Papi, Bella, Divina, and Stephen. You mean everything to me!

Of course, the one, the only, Sheri Hunt! For turning my jumbled thoughts into English.

Susan and Becky for their amazing editing skills.

Jeanette Dillard for the incredible cover art (including the impeccable sketch of my beloved Trix-C). You took my vision and put it on paper.

Ben Mayer, great job on formatting the cover. You got skills!
Thank you, Sharon Green for writing the beautiful foreword. You have blessed me.

Ooh, and I can't forget my personal office: The Loft Coffeehouse!

Pastor Scott Heare and Pastor John Hinkebein your sweet words always encourage me.

And the list goes on and on and on... I wish I could name you all here, but you know who you are!

Thank you!!

A Note to Readers

Throughout this book you'll see a variety of famous quotes, Bible verses, and thoughts from some of my closest friends and family. A lot of these famous quotes have inspired me to be who I am today. The Bible verses guided me through some rough experiences in life. Sheri and I were able to interview just a few of my family and closest friends to get their perspective on what it is like to live with someone with a disability.

A PARADOX OF VICTORY

CO-AUTHOR'S NOTE

Our writing group sat together in a cozy farmhouse living room, each huddled over notebooks and laptops. Trying to recall childhood memories drew us into individual cocoons of introspection.

When the front door opened, the production of wheelchair moving from outside to in was not really what diverted my attention. It was the hair. And the socks. And the smile. I'm not sure which was the first clue that this girl was going to be important in my life. Then she said, "I've always wanted to write a book."

That was when I knew.

A year passed before we met again. And from that day, The Loft Coffeehouse in Bulverde, Texas, became our office/conference room for the next two years as Nissi, the potential writer, became an author. To say this book has been a labor of love is correct. Any book is a laborious love-hate relationship with words, story crafting, editing, ad nauseum. But for me, personally, this journey has been about discovery, admiration and friendship.

Labor? Yes.

Love? YES!

You can't sit with Nissi for more than five minutes without someone saying to her, "You are so amazing." It's almost a joke how amazing she is and how often she hears it. I often tease her, "You will never hear those words from me. I don't want you to get a big head!"

But I think it all the time. ALL THE TIME. And it's not just the smile and the attitude: It *is* the wheelchair and the challenges it represents. The physical, mental, emotional toil it exacts. And the way this pink-haired beauty meets the challenges head-on like a football linebacker pushes those big padded machines on the practice field. The girl is fierce!

But more than anything (more than respect or admiration or wonder) what I really have gained over the last two years is a friend. A rare, real, true friend. A heart friend. We have learned from each other and grown as people through our friendship. If you are really lucky, this might happen only a handful of times in a lifetime.

In interviewing Nissi's friends and family for this book, one theme emerged: Nissi's strength comes from Jesus Christ. He is her rocket fuel as she charges into her full-speed-ahead, no-holds-barred, just-watch-me life. Nissi is happiest when her hair is blown straight back and bugs are hitting her teeth.

But her soul thrills in her Savior. And as I sat with her week after week talking about the people you will meet in these pages, I caught a glimpse of Jesus in this spazzy, jazzy girl in a wheelchair. I hope you will, too.

-SHERI HUNT-

FOREWORD

When I met Nissi, she always had a smile on her face and a kind word for everyone. It was the beginning of her junior year of high school and she was in my discipleship group at church. Like many teens, Nissi was battling to gain her independence, be a free thinker, outspoken, searching for her identity, tired of school, and ready for the future, though uncertain of what it held. But I quickly learned that behind the smile Nissi was trapped.

Every day was a reminder of just how different she was and the things that her life would never be. You see, Nissi was in a wheelchair, unable to care for herself - the constant reminder that she was different. The belt that held her in her chair was like a vice grip slowly crushing the life out of her. As much as she loved her twin sister, she was the reminder of what Nissi could never do.

She despised her chair, herself, and the constant reminders of how different she was. She was a captive who needed freedom.

Through real relationship and prayer, I began to see a hope replace the veil that had clouded her existence. Over the next few years as Nissi's heart healed and her confidence grew, she was willing to be vulnerable and tell her story.

She began inviting questions and conversation about the chair that she had long despised. She encouraged people to ask questions and found out that it really helped people to be comfortable. Their curiosity quickly turned from the chair to the person because Nissi is magnetic. People just want to be with her.

And after you've been around her, you find that you like life a little more, because she has rubbed off on you. She learned that she *was* different, but she was also really normal. Her contagious optimism balanced by the dose of reality that she cannot escape makes you realize your life, no matter how hard, can be blessed and fruitful. She is a picture of the healing and hope that Jesus brings. And she boasts in Him in everything - and sometimes uses words to do it. I have truly seen and tasted that the Lord is good.

It is rare to find people, especially younger people, who have a sense of self that is rooted in the truth of the gospel, and not some man-made impish version of the person they truly long to be. I have told my son that if there is one gift I could give him besides knowing Jesus, it's the gift of being comfortable in your own skin. Today, I find sitting before me a woman who has learned just that - Nissi is comfortable in her own skin. She has peace in the midst of the storms of life.

Not much about her daily routine has changed in the last 10 years. Nissi still uses a wheelchair to navigate the world. But her spirit soars free, unbound by the heartaches of life. Her smile can defeat the darkest heaviness, and the light in her eyes is warm and reminds you of what home should be.

I have watched Nissi shed the "tough girl" image for a healed heart. She no longer needs to put on the persona to be tough because she really is tough. Her vulnerability to live out her faith in Jesus (and be as kind to herself as He would) has made her a force to be reckoned with. I invite you to journey into the pages of Nissi's story and her heart to encounter the raw and the real - love, encouragement, healing and the Source of her eternal hope.

-Sharon Green-

A PARADOX OF VICTORY

table of contents

Heaven's Very Special Child

A meeting was held quite far from earth
"it's time again for another birth"
said angels of the Lord above.
"This special child will need much love,
her progress may seem very slow,
accomplishments she may not show,
and she'll require much extra care
from all the folks she meets down there.
She may not run or laugh or play.
Her thoughts may seem quite far away.
In many ways, she won't adapt.
And she will be known as handicapped.
So let's be careful where she's sent.
We want her life to be content.
Please, Lord, find the parents who
will do this special job for you.
They will not realize right away
the leading role they're asked to play.
But with the child from above.
Comes stronger faith and richer love
and soon they'll know the privilege given
in caring for this gift from heaven.
Their precious child so meek and mild
is **"heaven's very special child."**

Edna Massionilla

A PARADOX OF VICTORY

1. BEHIND THE SMILE, BEYOND THE CHAIR

She doesn't have an offense button, but she won't allow you to treat her like anything but her peer. That's her first superpower. Her other superpower is her hair.
—Scott— (Pastor)

By looking at me, you would never guess I'm in pain. In fact, my pain level is usually between a seven and an eight most of the time. For a month, I had a fractured ankle and didn't even know because of the level of pain I live with daily. Add to that, the discomfort of sitting on my bony booty hour after hour. My power chair is tolerable, but the manual chair feels like sitting on a hard-wooden bench. All. Day. Long.

✝

1

People provide wonderful distractions from this constant battle. When I spend time with people, I'm "up" and all smiles. But when I get home, I'm completely exhausted.

In public, I work hard to control the relentless spasms, which can occur four times each half hour. If you see me sitting on my hands or holding them down in my lap, you can pretty much assume I am fighting a silent battle with my arms. Silent on the outside. Screaming on the inside- because trying to control the floppy-like-a-drunk-marionette spasms only intensifies the existing pain.

Even without the spasms, I have a hard time keeping my legs still. They jerk around like a spider skittering back and forth. When my brain tries to cooperate, sometimes my body rebels. For instance, I have been known to kick people in the head who are just trying to get me into a car.

My brain and my body don't coexist harmoniously. They spend all my waking moments contradicting each other. Like a computer connected to a modem with a super glitchy connection.

When I was nineteen years old, I enrolled in a brain "boot camp." There, a brain specialist informed me that only 5% of my brain was working (compared to the normal range of 30%). According to the scans, I should not have been able to function. The doctor still cannot explain how I am able to talk.

For two weeks at camp, my brain endured 5-6 hours of daily stimulation exercises: Follow a ball with one eye and say a letter; crawl around like a sloth; jump on a trampoline. I'm not gonna tell you how that looked. I'm sure I smelled like a walking herb garden, since part of the therapy was being massaged with essential oils every hour. Detox diet. Constant activity.

The good news: The effort paid off with a 3% improvement in brain activity. I became more engaged, more active, as I grew stronger physically and mentally. The not-so-good news: If I don't use a skill on a daily basis, it gets lost in the mix.

Like Math. When I was younger, I was really good at math. But, when school ended, I stopped doing it. So that ability is gone. Without daily stimulation, I doubt that I will ever remember 8x7.

I can sit up, unaided, for an hour. According to the doctors, I shouldn't be able to do this. It does not make logical sense based on my brain scans. But that's half the fun of being me: If you tell me I can't, I'll show you that I can!

The only explanation for these illogical, science-defying abilities is they are gifts from God. He uses the foolish things of the world to confound the wise. He took a girl with Cerebral Palsy, placed her firmly in a wheelchair, and stuffed a defiant "stick-it-to-the-man" attitude in her rebellious body. That girl climbed Enchanted Rock, explored National Forests, and ran the Tough Mudder.

With a learning disability, I read at a 6th grade level. So, of course, I am writing a book. That makes perfect sense.

All my life, I have had neurological processing problems. For most of my life, my sister, Bella, spoke for me or translated my gibberish into functional words. But on the ride home from brain boot camp, I knew I wanted to be a motivational speaker. And I AM!

Because of the Lord Jesus Christ in my heart, I am a powerful woman. People think I am amazing. I know, because they tell me all the time. ALL THE TIME!

If I am amazing, it is because people see what I want them to see. It's my job. My purpose is to be a light no matter how I feel. It's not a luxury. It's a responsibility that sometimes stinks like a sewer! I can't be the way I want to be. I am a woman with fears and insecurities. I'm hormonal. Temperamental.

But in spite of all those roadblocks, I am a woman of great joy, surprising strength, and growing faith. In my life, I have learned to receive and give blessings. Inspire and be inspired. Accept compassion and praise. And exceed the limitations put on me by a medical diagnosis.

As for the future, it shouldn't surprise anyone that I want it all: Husband... children (yes, I can!)... a ranch in the

A PARADOX OF VICTORY

Texas Hill Country... travel as a motivational speaker...

climb mountains (oh yeah, been there, done that!) ...

...Visit Yosemite again.

I don't coddle her for any reason. I treat her like I treat everyone else. When I carry her, she tries to make me feel guilty, and I tease her about how heavy she is. But she's really a lightweight.
—Ben— (Close Friend)

✝

2. FIRST IMPRESSIONS

Seeing other people interact with Nissi, I learned people can smile and yet be ugly at the same time.

—Scott— (Pastor)

People react differently when they first meet me. Some smile immediately. Some sort of frown at first, followed by a smile. The third response is one of pure shock.

Most people smile, usually because I am smiling at them. I've been told many times I have a welcoming presence, and I draw people in with my smile. Those who start out with a frown are probably trying to figure out what's wrong with me. If someone doesn't see my chair, they are taken aback when they see that I need help to eat or drink. They seem a little confused, because I look pretty normal. Then they see someone helping me eat or drink and realize I have a disability. And sometimes that brings a smile of understanding my situation.

The people who show total shock see how comfortable I am with myself, and they don't know how to respond. My abrupt, sassy, outgoing, loud, and sarcastic comments surprises some people. My humor helps others realize I'm happy, just like I am.

My mom has a wild sense of humor, too. She's way out there, constantly making fun of herself, making us laugh at ourselves. I guess I get it from her: I'm always laughing and I like to make people feel comfortable.

I tend to discern when someone is wondering what's wrong. I just start talking. "Hi, my name is Nissi." I don't allow them to wonder if my brain works right and I want them to know I CAN talk. I try to be engaging as much as possible, so they don't have time to think about my disability. Instead of waiting for questions, I just tell them to get over it. I have.

My family taught me to not look at my disability as a disadvantage, but as a blessing. Because I am in a wheelchair, I can reach people that are intimidated or scared and make them feel comfortable with themselves. Even with me.

Who is Nissi Salazar?
Who am I?

I am Luis and Nancy Salazar's second oldest daughter. I am also a girl in a wheelchair. That's not what you want to know, is it? I bet you want to know that I'm a twin. Or is that not it either?

Oh, I see now! You want to know about what I have done, and who I am as a person. Well, warts and all, here we go:

In a family of four children, I was the third. I'm also the only disabled child. Some of you know what that means -

✝

I got away with everything. I was the queen at wiggling my way out of trouble. I was also born with a smile on my face. My mom said when my sister and I were about three months old, she went to check up on us at 3 a.m., and I looked up at her with the biggest smile on my face.

Hobbies? I have so many! I love people, animals and nature. I love fishing, horseback riding and dog training. I'm also a sucker for Broadway musicals. My two favorites are Phantom of the Opera and Les Misérables.

You could say I'm a modern-day Pocahontas with short hair (usually a different shade of purple, or pink, or blue). As you will find in this book, I am an adrenaline junkie - the faster, the better.

So, buckle my seatbelt, hold on tight, and LET'S GO!

Nothing gets her down. She is going to not let anything affect her. You can really tell the difference between people who feel bad for her and those who see the real Nissi. Passing strangers or those who know her and those who have sympathy, if others could see who she really is. But sometimes, people are so ignorant, I want to punch them in the face.

-Ben- (Close Friend)

A PARADOX OF VICTORY

✝

3. Overcoming Anxiety

The steadfast love of the Lord never ceases; his mercies never come to an end; they are new every morning; great is your faithfulness. "The Lord is my portion," says my soul, "therefore I will hope in him."

–Lamentations 3:22-24 ESV–

For three years, I fought an ongoing battle with myself and the enemy. It didn't matter if I **knew** the truth or not, uninvited fear always came. **Believing** the truth. That helped me conquer anxiety.

I don't remember when I started fighting for my freedom - freedom from my mind and from the enemy's poisonous words. All I can recall is I felt hopelessly trapped by my emotions. When the enemy started throwing lies at me:

"You are all alone. Everyone has forgotten about you. You will always be alone," I couldn't turn it off.

So, I started focusing on the truth, "My God will never leave me nor forsake me." I said these words over and over again. Then, I found power to say, "No," to the enemy every time he tried to flood my mind.

The whispers of the Father became battle cries. The enemy started to see me as someone not to be messed with, because I defied him with the most powerful truth, The Word of God!

When I was a young child, my mother forced me to recite scripture. At the time, I hated it. It wasn't until later, when anxiety attacks started at fourteen-years-old, that I truly appreciated my mother's persistence. She taught me that the Word of God is the sword of the Spirit. And I can tell you firsthand, it's very true.

One Scripture my mother made me recite when I was about eight years old is Psalm 91 (NIV):

1 Whoever dwells in the shelter of the Most High

A PARADOX OF VICTORY

will rest in the shadow of the Almighty.
I will say of the Lord, "He is my refuge and my fortress,
my God, in whom I trust."
Surely he will save you
from the fowler's snare
and from the deadly pestilence.
He will cover you with his feathers,
and under his wings you will find refuge;
his faithfulness will be your shield and rampart.
You will not fear the terror of night,
nor the arrow that flies by day,
nor the pestilence that stalks in the darkness,
nor the plague that destroys at midday.
A thousand may fall at your side,
ten thousand at your right hand,
but it will not come near you.
You will only observe with your eyes
and see the punishment of the wicked.
If you say, "The Lord is my refuge,"
and you make the Most High your dwelling,
no harm will overtake you,
no disaster will come near your tent.
For he will command his angels concerning you
to guard you in all your ways;
they will lift you up in their hands,
so that you will not strike your foot against a stone.
You will tread on the lion and the cobra;
you will trample the great lion and the serpent.
"Because he loves me," says the Lord, "I will rescue him;
I will protect him, for he acknowledges my name.
He will call on me, and I will answer him;

I will be with him in trouble,
I will deliver him and honor him.
With long life I will satisfy him
and show him my salvation."

In my younger years, I recalled this scripture from time to time, but it didn't have the same effect as when I started battling anxiety. Only then did I understand the full impact of those words. I started using the sword of the Spirit like never before. I fought the devil with my sword, the most powerful weapon in the universe. Who would have thunk the girl who cannot control her own body learned how to control her own mind.

I would love to tell you that I am completely healed. But the truth is, I am still fighting the enemy daily. But I have hope when my physical body gets tired or worn out, my spiritual body is strong in the Lord.

The best example I can think of, is the difference between using my power wheelchair versus my manual wheelchair. With my power chair, I feel physical freedom, like the sword of the Spirit gives spiritual freedom.

Almost every year on my birthday, I experience an anxiety attack. But the Lord is right beside me helping conquer the voices in my head. Even though my battle continues, I choose to believe the truth about what the Lord says- about who I am.

I am whole.

"Hardships often prepare ordinary people for an extraordinary destiny..."

~CS Lewis~

Fundamental truth about her: Without Christ she is unable to do anything. Not about what people affirm – it is about Christ within her. The Lord within her gives her strength and determination not found wholly within herself. It is her personality to be strong, but when her personality fails, Christ is there. Christ lifted her up in moments when she could not lift herself up. Yes, she rises above adversity, working hard. But, does that make her greater than other people? She is making a choice like everyone else can. We are all capable of overcoming. She is extraordinary, simply to make choices to overcome, but you can, too. Her disability brings that mindset of making wise choices to the front. She gets a lot of recognition and affirmation, but if she believes her own press, she will fall to a place of emptiness. If her value and worth is based on her ability and affirmation, that's not NISSI. I do think she is extraordinary, but only because of Christ in her.

–Bella– (Sister)

4. I AM HEALED

"It's wonderful to climb the liquid mountains of the sky. Behind me and before me is God and I have no fears."

-Helen Keller-

For as long as I can remember, people have been praying for my healing. I do believe one day the Lord will heal me. But that day might not be today or tomorrow. It's taken me a long time to realize who I am in Christ. The Lord created me to use my disability as a way to share his goodness and grace to the world. And when I discovered my destiny, I never wanted to let go. John 9 says it best:

"Now as Jesus was passing by,
he saw a man who had been blind from birth.
His disciples asked him,
"Rabbi, who committed the sin

✝

*that caused him to be born blind, this man or his
parents?" Jesus answered,
"Neither this man nor his parents sinned,
but he was born blind so that the acts of God
may be revealed through what happens to him.
We must perform the deeds of the one who sent me
as long as it is daytime.
Night is coming when no one can work."
9:1-4 John NET*

When I first heard this scripture, I immediately thought, *YES! This is who the Lord has made me to be. He created me to be his banner. For goodness sake, everybody already stares at me, why not use that for the glory of God?*

But unfortunately, not everybody sees it the way I see it. I've had so many reactions from people when they hear me say, "I don't think I'm supposed to get healed anytime soon."

I've heard, "You just have to have a little faith," and, "Well, don't you want to get healed?" I've lost count of how many people have prayed for me and expected results. Sometimes, I'm able to explain my viewpoint, but other times they just won't hear it. They don't understand that more often than not, my struggle is with my mind - not my body.

But then there are the beautiful few who see past my wheelchair and see me. These people pray for my heart and my inner man. Not just for my physical body. So many people don't realize before you can heal your body you have to heal your mind. Joni Eareckson Tada says this:

"It's not that Jesus didn't care about all those people it's just that their problems, especially their physical problems, weren't his main focus. The Gospel was his focus. The Gospel says: Sin kills, Hell is real. But God is merciful. His kingdom can change you and I am your passport."

In dark times, she gets overwhelmed by her life. Faced with daily and life-long limitations. We can never say to her, "If I was you." We cannot bridge that gap.

-Scott- (Pastor)

I learned a couple of things: need for community for wholeness AND development of who we are in our spiritual journeys - Physical and spiritual overlap. Nissi gives people eyes to see the spiritual underbelly. Physically it looks like she needs help. But spiritually she reminds us that we are all created for community, because we all have spiritual boundaries.

-John H- (Pastor)

5. MY FRAUD STATUS

Nissi actually changes the way you see physically challenged people for the rest of your life. You are curious about who they are as PEOPLE. You discover the treasure. You are willing to buy the field. You are willing to take all the field. You can see the kingdom of heaven is in her.

—Scott— (Pastor)

We all have those lies in our head. If you think you don't, I'm sorry to tell you, but you're not human. It's a fact of life. We all struggle, we all battle some kind of lie or disbelief.

For me, it sounds like: *You'll never be capable of being a motivational speaker.*

I'm an advocate for people with disabilities. I know the value of being transparent with people. But, in spite of those accomplishments, despite people telling me how amazing I am... I feel like a fraud most of the time. A fraud!

The lies continue based on these arguments:

- I have no business being a motivational speaker.
- I don't have a degree, I barely have a high school education.
- I have no business telling people what they should or shouldn't do with their lives.
- I can barely deal with my own crap!

Am I really happy all the time? Absolutely not.

Do I feel like I have to put on a show for everyone? Most days!

I believe the lie that I need to be on point all the time. I'm supposed to be setting a beautiful example of my heavenly father. I'm supposed to be setting an example for my family along with the disabled community.

Nissi is not allowed to feel broken or tired. Nissi is not allowed to be alone in a crowd full of people. I am the girl in the wheelchair who always has a smile on her face. I am not allowed to be hormonal or snappy. These are all extremely unrealistic things for a girl like me to carry on her shoulders alone.

But I do. In front of people, I tend to be this well-put-together girl, but when things start overwhelming me, the first people I attack are the ones that help me the most - my mom, my sisters, my dad, and my attendants. But the days which start with me snapping at my mom, or the others who have to help me on a daily basis, are the days I realize how solitary I make myself.

When I'm at my wits end, I start getting angry at myself for being so angry, I go outside and start yelling at the sky and the chickens: "Lord, THIS IS SO UNFAIR! Why me!? Why me?! Why couldn't I be someone else. Someone else to carry on your will... to bear this cross of disability!"

It's always a quiet Voice, it's always a patient Voice, when the Lord tells me, "You are not alone my Nissi. I have been here the whole time. Waiting for you to call me. I walk before you, next to you, behind you, and have been doing so your entire life. I haven't gone anywhere, and I will never leave you. Rely on me, and you can do anything! Let's show the world, my Nissi, what you can accomplish when you fully rely on me. Don't hold back, don't back down! My will be done in your life. You are perfectly imperfect."

So, do I accept my fraud status? Absolutely not! My mother reminded me about something the other day. Just because we feel a certain way or act a certain way doesn't mean it's who we are. I was made perfect in my weaknesses! Lies can come at me left and right, but, at the end of the day, I am so sure of who I am, because my heavenly father would never let me Forget! Please, don't forget who you are. You are beautiful, brilliant, talented and made perfect in his eyes. And let's be honest that's all that matters.

"Our deepest fear is not that we are inadequate, our deepest fear is that we are powerful beyond measure. It is our light, not our darkness, that most frightens us. We ask ourselves, who am I to be brilliant, gorgeous, talented, fabulous? Actually, who are you not to be? You are a child of God. Your playing small doesn't serve the world. There's nothing enlightened about shrinking so that other people won't feel insecure around you. It's not just in some of us; it's in everyone. And as we let our own light shine, we unconsciously give another people permission to do the same. As we are liberated from our own fear, our presence automatically liberates others."

-Marianne Williamson-

Nissi herself and her condition is a gift of God, but victory doesn't look like this, right? I have learned to know the meaning of "sufficient for the day is the evil thereof". Today I have enough grace. I live for today. I cannot worry about tomorrow or the next day. The reality is there is a whole world of suffering and imperfect people. Now I am part of that world and that world is part of me. It is a journey full of fighting.

-Nancy- (Mother)

6. CONTROL

But those who wait for the LORD's help find renewed strength; they rise up as if they had eagles' wings, they run without growing weary, they walk without getting tired.

—Isaiah 40:31 NET—

I love NOT being in control of my own life!! No, no, no... That's not right. Let me try again:

I am *learning* how to love not being in control of my own life!

I know, that's pretty funny coming from someone in my situation. Here is the truth: I decide what I wear, eat and who I see. I also decide where I go. But I have never truly felt like I was in control.

✝

Even though I decide what I wear, someone still has to dress me. I may decide what I eat, but someone still has to feed me. If I want to go out with friends, I always have to make sure someone's there who can physically pick me up or drive my car.

But let me tell you something: I have had some of the funniest conversations with my helpers getting dressed in the morning. And it's pretty hilarious when I'm riding with friends, and they're yelling at me from the back of their vehicle asking me how to tear apart my chair. The brave few who have driven my car? it's always an adventure!!!

When my dad feeds me, he sometimes brags about how great he is at feeding me. That makes me smile, because we have differing opinions. (Just kidding, Daddy!)

Not having control over certain situations has given me the opportunity to enjoy life in a whole new way. Like the time I had to go with my parents to their marriage retreat. Imagine a group of ultra conservative couples wondering why is this single girl, in a wheelchair, with

PURPLE hair doing at OUR marriage retreat? With a DOG?

I had to learn to laugh at times like this. I am not amazing at it! Actually, I probably suck at it. And that, my friends, is where the Big Guy Upstairs comes in. I could try all day long not to micromanage my life, but I'm only human, and humans tend to make mistakes. Some more than others.

Thank you Lord that your love and grace always covers me, and in you there is no guilt or shame!

The world does not revolve around how cute Nissi is. She's not all that special; Nissi is a brat.

—Bella— (Sister)

✝

I've learned that when you try to control everything, you enjoy nothing.

-LULU-

7. MY KINGDOM

Each time he said, "My grace is all you need. My power works best in weakness." So now I am glad to boast about my weaknesses, so that the power of Christ can work through me.

−2 Corinthians 12:9 NLT−

A lot of people don't know I was born in the East Coast. I'm a Texas girl through and through, but apparently, I'm also an East Coast girl. When I was three years old, my parents decided to move back to the great big state of Texas. I recall my mom telling me it was a very "Salazar" move. Which means, they kinda just left Maryland and didn't look back.

The first summer we spent in our single-wide mobile home, I remember all the exciting new smells and sounds. It was music to my ears even as a three-year-old. But, talk about hot and humid! And little to no running water. Not fun!

As a young kid, I never experienced the luxuries of having orange juice and apple juice or chips and candy for snacks. But, nevertheless, to me our home was the greatest place on earth. The most beautiful experiences I've had with my father God has been in the great outdoors of our property. Many times, when anger overwhelmed me, I could literally, and loudly, call out to God to heal my emotions. And he did. He brought peace into my angry soul, and joy into my pain-filled body. Being outside in the Texas Hill Country brought an overwhelming, satisfying feeling of freedom from everything but God and myself!

Before high school, I could wander around our whole property with a blindfold on and be perfectly fine. There wasn't a spot on our land I didn't know. When I was a kid, my mom would tell me to go outside and play. I would be gone for hours and hours. Back then, I didn't have a phone, so my mom had to come looking for me, and, more often than not, I was stuck somewhere.

This was almost a daily occurrence for me. I used to make up stories and go exploring with my dogs. Our property became my kingdom for adventure and fairytales. And as I got older, it became more and more of an escape. An escape from the yelling and the tantrums of normal household living. An escape from the pain that my body was enduring.

The trees became my jars of clay and I sculpted them bare. I used to strip the trees of bark, and mark them with a butter knife. Back when my little sister, Divine, used to actually listen to me, I used to make her dig me holes and see how far we (she) could dig without hitting a rock. These are the things we did for fun in my great kingdom.

I can't recall when it happened, but sometime between middle school and high school, I realized how small my castle and kingdom were. You see, my kingdom is 3 acres and my castle is still the single-wide mobile home. But by God's divine grace, knowing how small my kingdom was didn't affect how much I loved it. I'm not ashamed of it. In fact, I grew to respect it more and write many blog posts about this little place of refuge.

Amongst any chaos, I still have my little kingdom. A place where I can go wandering and feel as young as I once was.

In this little home, I learned how to love others, be respectful and, most importantly, how to be humble. Now that I'm older, I've had opportunities to stay in homes of all shapes and sizes. I've had the opportunity to stay in places where the apple juice and orange juice are overflowing, but every time, I miss my home. I miss the simplicity of the beautiful place I call my castle!

"The Word gave life to everything that was created, and his life brought light to everyone. The light shines in the darkness, and the darkness can never extinguish it."

John 1:4-5 NLT

"...Like standing on the edge
Of a mountainside
I can feel the wind stirring
Lifting me up high
I was born into freedom
I was made to fly..."

—Catch the Wind,
Jonathan David & Melissa Helser—

8. My Heroes

Make sure you don't take things for granted and go slack in working for the common good; share what you have with others. God takes particular pleasure in acts of worship—a different kind of "sacrifice"—that take place in kitchen and workplace and on the streets.

—Hebrews 13:16 MSG—

Besides my parents, my one brother and two sisters have felt the full brunt of my disabilities. But the Lord knew exactly what I needed in siblings.

The oldest of the four is my brother, Stephen. Stephen is five years older than us twins. Stephen, a genius in my eyes, usually excels at anything he tries, whether it be music or mechanics. On many occasions I honestly thought my brother would've made an excellent CIA agent.

Isabel (who we all call Bella) is 24 minutes older than me. Bella, one of the most understanding and nurturing people I know, knows how to say things eloquently and with conviction. Just like Stephen, she is musically talented. They both sing and play their instruments with such passion. But, despite all her caring and nurturing, Bella could be an assassin. You do not want to cross that girl!

And then there's Divine Grace who is wise beyond her years! Divine could just rule the world, because she has never met a child or animal that does not love her! She has a gentle but assertive way of handling children and animals that makes them want to flock to her.

Naturally, my parents focused on me instead of prioritizing my brother and sisters. No handbook existed on how to handle a child with a disability who had siblings, so they did the best they could.

But I knew Stephen, Bella and Divine resented me. For example, in third grade, Bella was invited to a slumber party. I was not.

"I'm going," I announced.

Bella panicked. "Please, please, don't make me bring her!"

"I'm going!" I stated emphatically, before I launched into a fit.

I saw Bella crumble before my eyes. From that time on, a little piece of Bella died every time my parents allowed her to go, but not spend the night because of me.

On the other hand, Stephen actively included me at all costs. My brother was my biggest bodyguard growing up, protecting me from loneliness, even at the expense of others.

When I was three, my mom was videotaping me crawling on the floor. She wanted to show my physical therapist how I moved around our home, but the video captured a bigger drama:

Bella wanted to put on a puppet show. When Stephen took over, Bella threw a tantrum.

✝

"No Bella," Stephen said.

"No, Bella," I repeated like a trained parrot.

"Let Nissi play."

"Let Nissi play."

Stephen dragged me to the puppet show, and kicked Bella out, which started one of her legendary tantrums, screaming and falling to the ground to wail more! Poor Bella. Not only did we steal her puppet show: She got in trouble for throwing a fit.

As for Divine, she could never comprehend why I got special treatment. From the beginning, she wanted me to "get over it." She still has a hard time understanding how I meet challenges differently from her. But she is valuable in my life. From her, I learn to walk in blunt truth. From me, she can learn to react with compassion. We are still on the journey of appreciating our differences.

My siblings and I were with each other almost 24 hours a day, till Stephen started going to public school his senior year. We learned so much in our tiny home. Over the years, our parents raised us to love and respect each other no matter what. The Salazar household had a strict "no-name-calling" policy.

I live continually amazed at how strong the Lord has made my brother and sisters. I see where they are today, and it blows my mind.

Even now, when I am with my brother, he still tries to protect me from the stares of curious people. He has a beautiful way of speaking to people with disabilities with the same respect he demands for me, his little sister! His protective nature to defend those in need has gotten him in and out of trouble, but it has also made him fearless! For example, Stephen was at a party with a group of friends and he saw a guy mistreating his girlfriend. Without even thinking, my brother pommeled the guy to the ground.

As for my sweet Bella, even now, I'm writing this in tears. Bella is the most beautiful person inside and out. Growing

43

up with her was like watching a rose blossom for the first time. Her strength has carried many people through hard times. She understands when no one else does, because she has had to pick herself off the ground so many times. She is the "Mother Theresa of Tomorrow" in my book!

Like my big brother and twin sister, Divine is extremely strong in her own way - the most fierce and badass of the four of us. Earlier this year, when I did the Tough Mudder, she very adamantly kept reminding me to drink water, at times shouting and shoving the water in my face to keep me hydrated. This is who she is - she protects those in her corner like a vicious lioness.

When I asked my brother, "What did you learn from living with me, someone with a disability?"

On the other end of the phone, he snorted and said, "Sis, we're *still* learning how to live with someone with a disability." My sisters and I would agree. No, we do not have this down to a science. But, oh, how far we have come!

Families are the compass that guides us. They are the inspiration to reach great heights, and our comfort when we occasionally falter."

—Brad Henry

9. BELLA

Nissi is not all that and a bag of chips.
—Bella— (sister)

Bella and I have known each other since conception! Before I thought my first thought, she was there. Before we cried for the first time, we were together.

Even though we haven't known anything else, we still marvel at this fact of our life. We were one, and became two. Are we one person? No. We are two individuals, vastly different, that started life as one single egg.

It's only natural we are closer and know each other better than everyone around us. As little girls, we shared a queen-size bed. When a storm woke us in the middle of the night, Bella held my hand and told me everything was gonna be alright. Then she dragged me on a towel across our house to camp out at the door of our parents' room. I'm sure we were quite a sight.

As we grew, it became obvious Bella was the more dominant twin. When we played, she was the mother, and I was the daughter. My mom tells the story: "Nissi would say, 'Mama. Mama,' and I would respond, but she was actually talking to Bella."

The older we got, Bella started taking the role of second mother very seriously. I don't think my parents meant to do this, but they unconsciously made Bella feel responsible for my happiness and well-being. They expected her to include me in whatever she did. She grew up constantly hearing, "Take care of your sister" and "Bella, why aren't you including your sister?" No 10-year-old little girl wants to feel like that.

I can almost guarantee my parents didn't mean to do this to their sweet little girl. But, unfortunately, that's exactly what happened. Bella had to grow up too fast, and she grew to resent me in the process. One of the most horrendous experiences for me was watching the light drain out of my twin sister's eyes during our childhood.

Luckily, us Salazar women are made of more leather than lace - we are a tough breed. My beautiful sister didn't let resentment cloud her love for me. She never let it affect our relationship, but continued to nurture and minister to me as a loving sister.

Bella remembers this story, which beautifully represents the responsibility and challenges we faced:

We were maybe fifteen-years-old and we were alone at home. Nissi started bouncing on the couch and yelling, 'I HAVE TO GO TO THE BATHROOM!'

Seeing her being bathed was normal. So, it was not weird helping her. But, even though I dragged her around the house on a towel since we were little, and even though I had helped my mom take her, I freaked out on how I was going to do this by myself. She is heavy! "Can you hold it till mom gets home?"

Still bouncing on the sofa, she squeaks out, "NO! I CAN'T HOLD IT! I HAVE TO GO NOW!"

Can I do this? I have to do this! "Okay! This is about to go down!"

I lifted her from the couch to the floor and dragged her by her arms down the hall to our really small bathroom in our really small mobile home.

About halfway there, we both start laughing. Somehow, we made it to the bathroom door. I pull her pants down, but we are laughing so hard, neither of us is sure if she is going to make it.

"Breathe," I manage to sputter between giggles.

I don't know how I managed to get her on the toilet, but we did. Disaster avoided.

Just one of our many stories. Writing all of them would take a whole book.

Growing up, I knew that I was the center of attention: I didn't know how not to be. Of course, she resented it, but I only knew how to care about myself and did not know how to get out of my selfishness. I blamed my parents for not paying attention to her, but she blamed me.

But we were all doing this for the first time – my parents, siblings and me. By the time we got to high school, my parents started prioritizing my siblings instead of just me. My brother and sisters still had to deal with feelings of jealousy from years of me taking so much of my parent's time and energy. Even though I knew Bella harbored deeply buried resentment towards me, she still managed to be completely loving, caring and compassionate towards me.

On the other hand, I did not handle my resentment of Bella as graciously.

As we got older, our differences became obvious. I did not like this, AT ALL!! We were twins, darn it! We were supposed to dress the same, act the same and look the same, right? Bella wanted to be a girly-girl, but I did not care about what I looked like or what I wore. She loved dresses, but I liked wearing pants with a bandana stuck on my head. No curls for me, please.

I didn't want to be noticed, and I thought the best way

to vanish was to be unnoticeable. I wanted to disappear behind her beauty. Fade into the background. Be eclipsed by her obvious loveliness. Good luck with that philosophy in a wheelchair. EVERYONE noticed me.

Around this time, my hair became my greatest experiment, and I embraced the reality that people did noticed me. I could not escape or just disappear. One day, at the hair salon Bella suggested that we get different hairstyles, for the first time in our lives. I got my hair colored dark red, and Bella got hers highlighted.

I ABSOLUTELY LOVED my hair. Bella hated hers. She vowed she would never color her hair again. I didn't understand why Bella didn't want to cut her hair as well. When Bella's hair started growing into her natural color, I urged her to color it again, but she never did! Well, at least she never highlighted it again. Me, on the other hand, I think I've colored my hair every shade of the rainbow possible. And I mean EVERY shade. Whether it be on purpose or not.

As identical twins, recognizing our differences built another dynamic into our relationship: Most people let me get away with a lot of crap, but I can't bullshit Bella. She is the only person on the planet who knows me inside and out. Like a fine-tuned machine, she knows my reactions and what I am going to say, even before I do. Sometimes I think she has fun challenging my brattiness.

For example, not long ago, my family wanted to go out to eat, and my taste buds were hungry for Olive Garden. As soon as we were loaded into the car, I start: "I want to go to Olive Garden."

My parents, who always try to accommodate me (I have programmed them well) start the car and head down the highway to warm bread sticks.

From the back of the car, little sister, Divine, says, "Chili's sounds good…"

Now the battle begins – the one that I am sure to win. While Divine makes her polite suggestion only once, I loudly and continually talk about how good Italian food is:

"Mom, remember they have that great salad at Olive Garden? Pasta is my favorite meal ever! And Dad loves those breadsticks." My mom starts to crumble without even knowing that I am completely manipulating the situation.

Meanwhile, Bella, a big old grin on her face, chimes in: "Nissi, didn't you just have pasta just a couple of days ago?"

Then my mom says, "Oh, that's right, we did have pasta just a couple of days ago."

I want to punch Bella's pretty little face. My plan was going so well.

We end up going to Chili's.

I wish I could stay mad at her, but the truth is there is no one else whose affection I crave more than Bella's. Even though she is the only person who can set me off from 0 to 100 on the angry scale in two seconds, I eagerly look forward to cuddle time on the sofa with my sister.

On the couch, I lean heavy against her, half of my body on her lap. She is on the phone with her boyfriend, but she strokes my hair. Although we do not manifest affection the same way (she is not a physical person), she does it for me. Nothing makes me feel more safe, more put together, completely and utterly whole. I am "at home" with Bella.

This is the part of her mothering instinct I love. And the fact that she helped me realize I am a brat and encouraged me to use my powers for good. But sometimes, I remind her she is not my mother. Like when she corrects me in front of people.

Bella has grown into accepting the attention that my wheelchair brings me. We make fun of it. For Christmas, we go shopping. The seas part. Handicap parking has its advantages!

Bella has taught me the value of compassion and sensitivity. She pays attention on purpose, because she cares and wants to help. She always knows the right thing to say and buys just the right gifts. She just knows people.

When Bella sings, she SINGS. Even though my brother is a musician, and I love his art, Bella's words and voice lifts up my heart like no other music. I feel her strength of emotion from every song.

I'd have to be dead not to be jealous of Bella: Exceptionally beautiful and able to say eloquent words in a second. Meanwhile, it takes me 15 minutes to figure out what to say in a phone conversation. She is musically gifted. Even if I could sing, I could not do what Bella does.

Our differences have given us advantages, as well.

The year the twin and I graduated high school, my parents gave us a gift: A trip to Colombia. Unfortunately, my dad had to work all summer long, so it was just Momma and us three girls who ventured to South America. As soon as they purchased the tickets, my mom started looking for exciting things for us to do while we were down there. After a few days of searching the interwebs, she found a

Christian camp coinciding with our trip. It didn't matter if we wanted to go or not, Momma decided Bella and I had to go.

Everyone forgot to mention that South Americans, for the most part speak only Spanish. We do not. Talk about culture shock. My mom forgot to tell the camp staff about the language barrier.

When we arrived at the church for the 5-hour bus ride to the camp, I watched the panic meter rise as the staff tried to get our medical history and information about how to care for me.

Eventually, we got everything covered and Momma left. I don't think she looked back once - we were in good hands and she was free! On the bus, Bella and I clung to each other with everyone chattering around us in Spanish or 2% English.

One girl decided she was going to break the language barrier. She was not going to let our fear or her lack of English stop her from making friends. Over the next few miles, we had a breakthrough that changed our whole camp experience.

As Spunky Colombian Girl tried to make conversation, I realized I could understand just enough to translate to Bella. Bella could speak just enough Spanish to reply. So Bella and I became one mechanism with just enough skill to turn what could have been a disastrous week into a miraculous time of beautiful interdependence. We needed each other to thrive. And we did!

Bella and I are alike, but different. Part of our path toward maturity has been that each of us must embrace our similarities and differences alike: She has learned to accept the fact that we are twins, and that she is stuck with me forever. I have learned that being a twin doesn't mean I have to be a leech.

We have learned to conquer jealousy and find security in how God created us so alike and so different at the same time. In loving my sister, I have learned that part of me is lovable, simply because I am so much like her. And I have learned to embrace those things which make us completely separate and unique.

She is genetically exactly the same as Bella – identical twin, same dynamic personality, drastically different physical challenges. How do they square this up with God?

-Scott- (Pastor)

I have a master's degree in NISSI. I know what she needs before most people. I can read her and predict her needs from her physical behaviors.

–Bella– (sister)

10. MOMMA

*...he is a product of her
upbringing: Her mom
relentlessly told her she was
...pable.*

—Ben and/or Scott and/or John—

"There is no one like your momma."

This cheesy saying couldn't be more true for me. I'm going to attempt to articulate the amazing woman who raised me. I doubt I will do her justice, but I will do my best.

But if a woman have long hair, it is a glory to her...
1 Corinthians 11:15 (KJV)

If that statement is true, my mom is the most glorious woman alive!

✝

One of the earliest memories I have of my mother is when I was 3 years old. Laying in her bed at night listening to her sing a lullaby inspired by Psalm 139:

I will praise you Lord,
for My Nissi was fearfully and wonderfully made.
I will praise you Lord,
for my Nissi was fearfully and wonderfully made.
Wonderful is my Nissi,
and that my soul knoweth well.
Wonderful is my Nissi,
and that my soul knoweth well!

The lullaby made me feel safe, warm and loved, even though she could not sing to save her life, it was beautiful to me.

There is no question I get my wild streak from her. When my mom was younger, she was the type of person who acted first and thought later. Quietly passionate and adventurous, my mom would take me with a group of kids, all under the age of 12, to the park. She encouraged her children to be adventurous and carefree. Momma didn't want us to live in fear of the unknown. The type of person who said, "We'll be fine." And we were.

Maybe you are wondering, "Wow, what was she thinking? Did she not care?" Actually, quite the opposite is true.

For as long as I have been alive, maybe even longer, my mother has relied FULLY on Jesus. It's not that she doesn't think about all the things that could go wrong. Believe me, she does. But her faith is enough to allow her children and herself to live completely free.

That is who my mother is at her core...faithful. Faithful to the Lord. Faithful to her husband and to her children. To this day, even though technically speaking she doesn't "parent" us anymore, she still guides us, sharing her wisdom. Before group texting and the GroupMe app, my mother daily sent all four of her children words of encouragement individually: Now she sends it in a group text! If one of us has some sort of issue, whether it be financial, physical or emotional, my mother is the first to offer prayer and advice.

My mom and I have a very special relationship. You could

say we were attached at the hip as I was growing up. I did everything with my Momma. If she went to Bible study, I tagged along. Homeschool parent meeting? I was there.

Even at home, she was my safe space for so many years. Still is. The first person I see when I wake up in the morning, and the last one I see when I go to bed. She is my personal stylist, hair colorist, dog training assistant and counselor.

There are so many layers to my mom: Wise and loving. Wildly free - like Hakuna Matata. But it's all based on her faith in the Lord.

Even when I was as young as six years old, Momma Bear encouraged me to go outside and run around by myself. She apparently didn't think about me for hours. Nonchalant - in a good way. Not a helicopter parent at all, in fact, I wonder if she realized I was disabled.

As soft-spoken and demure as she appears, on the inside the woman is a tom-boy! She often jokes that she should have been the mother of all boys. She loved us girls, but the boys liked climbing trees and digging in the dirt and trekking through the brushy hillsides.

She responded like most men would to an accident: "Did you break your arm? That's ok, honey. You're strong, go back outside and climb more trees." Of course, this is an exaggeration, but you get the idea.

For instance, when the youth pastor planned activities, he always called parents to let them know the driving arrangements - who was riding in whose car. Stuff like that.

When he called my mom to let her know whose car I would be in, she would say, "Fine. Whatever works." When they hung up, she said, "Tell John he doesn't have to call me with miniscule things. I don't need to know."

When I was 17, my dad hung a tarp strap in a tree. He called it a swing. My mom called it ghetto, hillbilly, and begged him to take it down. He was way too proud of that ugly thing. Years later, my mom got that look in her eye: "I'm gonna go get that ugly swing out of the tree."

"Mom! No, you are NOT! You'll fall and break your neck!

You can guess who won that argument. Macie took pics of mom swinging like Tarzan, her hair flowing free behind her.

Don't think for a minute she doesn't have a soft side. For example, she learned braille when I was 19. She loves blind people, and wanted to be a braille translator.

She always wanted to adopt another child. As if homeschooling four kids in a tiny house wasn't enough. As if a daughter in wheelchair didn't present enough challenges. She wanted to add another special needs child to the mix! To this day, she still talks about it. Sometimes I doubt her sanity. Fo' real!

She is so in tune with the Spirit of God and so solid in her faith, she makes pastors look like choir boys! If we are sick, we have no choice but to feel better with Momma. She speaks with power. Her presence radiates peace, grounding people with her sweet, gentle, firm spirit. That's how powerful her faith and mothering nature is.

Born into a family that suffers from depression, my mom escaped that curse. She lives beautifully carefree, but deeply caring. She is as untamed as her glorious mane. Yes, her hair can be controlled, but why mess with a good thing?

I hope to follow her example of quiet faith, risky adventure, and selfless love.

Momma tends to enable us, because she does everything! There are no boundaries – even if she is sick or dying, she will help Nissi. She is that way for anyone who needs help.

—Divina– (Sister)

Long ago the LORD said to Israel: "I have loved you, my people, with an everlasting love. With unfailing love I have drawn you to myself."

—Jeremiah 31:3 NLT–

Our life is boot camp. Nissi an extension of me. Connected in all ways. She needs my help physically so much, I feel like even when I am gone, I always have one foot at home. I have those moments when I look at her inabilities, all her friends and sisters, being able to do things. If I look and focus, it will consume me. I choose to not look at those things. I am her example. If I crumble, she crumbles. But she encourages me with her strength.

—Nancy— (Mother)

It was hard to grow up with Nissi. I was easily forgotten and neglected because I was easy. So, I resented that she was center of attention. My mom's full-time job was to focus on her. It didn't leave much time for the rest of us. Looking back, I see it all as the best learning experience. I learned anything is possible.

—Bella— (sister)

11. MI PAPI

"...You split the sea
So I could walk right through it
My fears were drowned in perfect love
You rescued me
And I will stand and sing
I am the child of God..."

-No Longer Slaves: Jonathan David &
Melissa Helser-

"God gave me a star. You know where it is?"

"In your arms!"

"That's right!"

For as long as I can remember, my dad and I have this conversation every time he carries me from car to the house. You could call it "our thing". Growing up with three siblings who were all talented in whatever they did, you can imagine what this did for my self-esteem.

✝

My father believes in his family with all of his heart! Whatever we do, he supports 110%. No joke! I have lost count on how many times my Dad has offered to both my musical siblings: "If you make me your manager, I'll make you famous in a heartbeat."

My ability to read people comes from my dad. But I also get my stubbornness and temper from my old man. Like many great men, my father struggled most of his life to be the man God created him to be. It's safe to say he's been to hell and back! For so many years, it was hard for me to understand why he lost control and got so angry. Why he would say such hurtful words to my mom and to us, his children?

I didn't understand psychological terminology like "orphan spirit" or "self-loathing". My daddy didn't know how to channel all the rejection and abuse he endured as a child. Not until he learned how to rely on God for absolutely everything! After discovering his identity in Christ, my father didn't feel like he had to shoulder all the pressure of being the perfect husband and father. He became free to just be himself.

I absolutely love when my father is just being himself! Goofy. Good with words. And the man knows how to dress! Passionate, devoted, hard-working, and totally in love with my mother. Even with all the crap that we went through when I was young, I wouldn't have chosen differently in the Papa Bear department.

He has so much to do with the way I feel for people and the reason I love so deeply. He's my heater in the winter and my personal tow truck. Like my mother, he believes in me and believes I can do anything I put my heart to do.

One of the favorite things about my amazing dad is hearing him share his heritage with people. My father is a proud Colombian Jew. Because of him, we went to a Messianic synagogue when I was little, and I know some Jewish prayers! I have such a huge heart for my Jewish heritage, and in case you didn't realize this, my name is

A PARADOX OF VICTORY

Hebrew for "victory/banner".

Sometimes, I forget I live with a living, breathing miracle. There's no other way to explain it, that's what my father is. A fatherless boy became a great father. God molded him right before my very eyes. God stripped him bare of the self-protective shield he wore to expose the big teddy bear I knew was always there.

From a home of neglect, he became a father who treasures his children. He sees us as destined for greatness and uses all his resources to help each of his children realize their own potential. Papi cheers us on as he watches his dreams and hopes fulfilled in what we do and who we are. For a man who lacked nurturing as a child, he has excelled at nurturing his own children with strength of character, stubborn determination, and great joy.

Papi was gone a lot. He's always liked to take Nissi places, but I never saw him helping much when she was little. Whenever he did something for her, he made a make a big deal about it: He wanted credit for "taking care" of Nissi! Later in life, he became more compassionate. Sometimes he treats her like she is gonna break.

-Divina- (Sister)

A PARADOX OF VICTORY

✝

12. STEPHEN

"Failures, repeated failures, are finger posts on the road to achievement. One fails forward toward success."
—C. S. Lewis—

The other day, as I was looking through family photos, I came across a photo that made me smile and tear up at the same time. In this photo, my brother is five-years-old holding his two newborn baby sisters with a big smile on his face.

"My life was never the same after that day," he jokes. In a matter of minutes, he went from being "number one son" to the older brother and the last to receive attention. I can only imagine how traumatic that must've been for a five-year-old used to getting all the attention from our parents and extended family. No longer the cutest thing around town. He got bested by, not ONE, but TWO little sisters. Maybe he could live with one, but two was not part of the deal.

I can't tell you what he was like those first few years. But I can say that for as long as I can remember, my big brother has always looked out for me. Besides Bella, he was my only friend for a long, long time.

The year he moved out of the house to the University of the Incarnate Word was beyond hard for me. I felt like my world was falling apart right before my eyes. I was thirteen when he moved to Boston. To this day, I don't think he knows how I stayed up for hours crying the morning he left. My hero was leaving me behind. I felt alone and betrayed. I thought no one would ever understood me as my free-spirited brother did. Every fiber of my being wanted to get in a suitcase and go with him. Even if he didn't want me!

As a young child, I wanted to be just like him. My brother was good at everything he did. He didn't care about consequences or, more importantly, didn't care what people thought of him. I wanted that freedom. I thought he could teach me how to be free. Free of my disability. Free of my insecurities, and free to be totally ME!

My lovely twin sister likes to tell me I am the most stubborn person she knows. I usually laugh, and she says, "Oh, that wasn't a compliment, my dear." I have to say, I'm afraid she's right. At least a little right. My stubborness is probably why it took me many years to forgive my brother for something he didn't have any control over.

Like I did with Bella, I made Stephen my God. But Stephen is only human. Humans are flawed and make mistakes. When he left, I thought my world was over. Who was going to teach me how to be free? Somehow, between the time I was thirteen to the time I was eighteen, I learned how to become my own person. Finally, I began to forgive my brother for leaving me. I started realizing who I was as a human being, as a child of God, and as someone with a disability.

Some of my best memories are with my brother. And, as hard as it is for me to admit it, my brother leaving home was probably one of the best things for me. I couldn't stay in his shadow forever.

Now, when Stephen comes home to visit, I treasure every moment I have with him. We laugh so much! My sisters and I agree vacations don't really start until he arrives. He always makes us feel like little girls again, and it's always bittersweet. If he comes home during the summer, it's been our tradition to go fishing together. Before he left home, if we ever went on a fishing trip at the coast, the girls always stayed on the beach, and my brother and parents would go with me deep-sea fishing. It's our thing!

Stephen also taught me how to play chess very well. I was eight years old. I knew how to play, but didn't know any of the chess piece names. He also taught me how to play poker and encouraged me to play the harmonica.

I think my brother saw that I was feeling left out of the recitals and the lessons, and so he taught me these things to help me cope with my disability. I think he wanted me to feel as though I could accomplish something - be good at something. Even though I don't play chess as well as I used to, anytime I do play, I smile, because no one thought I could play but my brother.

When my cousins play poker, I laugh, because I know how to play better than they do. Why? Because my brother wanted me to feel included. He still insists that I learn how to do things. Whether it be designing websites or creating electronic music on the computer, he's always encouraging me to go further. He even went so far as to tell me I could be a comedian.

"No way. No how, big brother," I told him!

Sometimes when I'm feeling blue, like I can't do anything, I remember the time Stephen went to Boston with only $50 in his pocket. If he could do that, I can do anything!

I love you, big brother!

I was like his child. Of all the siblings, we have always been the most comfortable with each other. He was the funny big brother. Bella had to grow up so fast — she had to take care of us, but Stephen took time to play with me.
—Divina— (Sister)

13. DIVINA

Ugh. ALL my friends love you.

-Divina-

I have a special relationship with Bella, because she's my twin. I have a special relationship with my brother because he's my only brother. I have extraordinary relationship with my little sister, because she is the one who never lets me forget that I'm normal. She is the one who would never allow me to be spoiled, selfish or full of myself.

Divine is seven years younger than me. Her gorgeous wild curly hair gave her the nickname of "Leona", which means lioness in Spanish. You couldn't write a better description of her. The girl is fierce.

Ever since she was a baby, Divine has never done anything half-ass. If she had a tantrum, it was a full-on meltdown. If she was happy, you couldn't stop her from smiling or laughing. For as long as I can remember, animals and babies flock to her. Her dominant personality attracts them. In fact, at the ripe age of five she would lead around our 1500-pound horse like he was a miniature pony.

It is by God's divine grace that Divine Grace is alive today. My mom got very sick when she was pregnant with my little sister. They both could've died. But Divine had the rough end of that stick. Divine was 11 weeks early and so tiny, my dad could hold her in one hand. A week after she was born, her tummy started turning a different color. At 2 lbs. 6 oz. they did two major surgeries on our little warrior. She wasn't supposed to survive either of them.

The Lord gave my mom Divine's name when she was born. But my mama was stubborn, she named her something else:

Grace Lynn. But, after those two surgeries Momma changed it to what it was supposed to be - Divine Grace - a constant reminder of God's intervention in their lives.

Because she was a preemie, she faces a unique set of ongoing challenges. Nothing like mine - she can walk, feed herself, drive. And the girl knows how to have fun. But sometimes, her amazing strength can be misinterpreted as aggression. Some people bring it out more than others. One of those people is yours truly.

One of my earliest memories is I was crawling on the floor, and she kicked me. Just flat-out punted me. She didn't understand why I couldn't move like she could, so she booted me out of the way.

To Divine everything is black or white. I live in the gray. So, that's what makes her extraordinary. Divine has values that will never be swayed by the world or the people around her. But this means she has limited empathy for someone, like me, who lives in constant battle with the norms of today's society.

Some of the many questions my little sister asks me in a frustrated voice is: "Why can't you move out of the house? Get a job?" I know what she's really asking, "Why won't you do something with your life?" She's not asking these questions to be harsh or condescending. It's just her way of caring for me.

Divine and I inherited our father's temper. So when we get into it, we really get into it! But I never want to hurt my baby sister, so I'm always the first to back down. I stole her childhood in so many ways: I will never be able to repay the things she had to sacrifice for her big sister.

I am overly aware of the sacrifices my family members had to make to have a disabled sister. I know it is not my job to try to heal wounds so deep only the Lord can heal, but I will do whatever is in my power to make them know that they are loved and valued!

Strong love looks different for many people: Even though we butt heads, our conflicts are rooted in a deep, heart-wrenching love. Her passion makes her speak the truth

100%. No diluting with nice words. Her concerns are that intense.

Divine gets exceptionally annoyed with me when I act like a complete brat and 10 minutes later I'm acting like an angel in front of friends or strangers. For example:

Let's say, my mom cooks something that I can't stand. This, of course, is a mortal sin, resulting in a complete pity party howling hissy fit.

Divine looks at me like I'm an alien and tells me as much. "Are you five?" She asks me with the most condescending and annoyed voice possible.

"Divine, don't talk to your sister like that!" Interjects my mom.

Once again, I start whining about the injustice of me not being able to eat something I like.

And say, after this whole conversation we decide to go to The Loft Coffee House. Upon arrival, I run in to friends who start telling me how wonderful and amazing I am. I glance at my wonderful little sister: Her eyes rolling back

50,000,000 feet! I know what she's thinking.

Fierce lioness in a small package.
Little do you know people! Little do you know!

"Doubt the stars are fire;
Doubt that the sun doth move;
Doubt the truth be a liar;
But never doubt I love."

-William Shakespeare-

People think she is not mentally there
because she is in a wheelchair and her
body does not move normally, so I had
higher standards for her. Because
mentally she is all there.

-Divina- (Sister)

14. THE SQUID

Generally, she is strong like a syrupy song. But if you pick on her, she can slap right back. Did I mention she is condescending? If pity sneaks into a sentence she will snip it out and burn you down.

—Scott— (Pastor)

People typically ask, "How is it that you're so good at giving as good as you get?" This is one of the funniest questions, because they're not talking about charity and/or giving back to the community.

Oh no, they're talking about my sassiness!

Sarcasm is my second language, and sometimes that scares people. They just don't get it. When I make fun of myself, maybe they're not sure how to take it. It makes them squirm a little, so to add fuel to the fire, I tease them.

✝

The answer to my quick with and sarcastic nature is plain and simple: "I was raised with a bunch of boys."

While it's true I only have one biological brother (who I swear equals four brothers), I come from a very large family. Of my cousins who live in Texas, there are six girls and eight boys in our crazy posse. The boys lived to tease the girls. They nailed our Barbie dolls to trees and beheaded them. They also called us wonderful nicknames like "Telephone Pole" and "Bigfoot". Many times, my precious sister, Bella, ran home crying, because the boys were being so mean to her. Even though Divine was their "Baby", she did not escape the torture. But, because she wanted to be one of the boys, she learned how to toughen up.

They were mean to me, too! Because I have cerebral palsy, my arms move and jerk all the time. So, one Christmas, they crossed out my name on the gift tags and wrote, "Squid". Of course, the name stuck. But, for some reason, the teasing didn't affect me the same way it affected my sister or my other girl cousins.

To be honest, sometimes I loved being tortured by the boys. Mainly, because I knew they didn't care that I was in a wheelchair. No sir! They refused to treat me like I had some sort of disease! Their favorite thing to do was unplug my wheelchair and leave me in the middle of the road. Terrifying, but so, so, so funny!

My cousins were the first ones who accepted me for me! Boys and girls alike taught me to look beyond insults and to not give a crap what other people think. Because of our relationship, I learned to be resilient and to give as good as I get! They taught me the importance of loyalty and family.

I taught them a thing or two, as well. From me, they learned the importance of a good attitude about life. And, they **had** to learn the responsibility of caring for others.

Eventually, we all grew up. Some of us even matured!

If you were to see us out and about, you might think we were all brothers and sisters. Maybe you will see my little sister sitting on one of my older cousin's lap. Or you'll see another cousin feeding me. To be honest, it's by the grace

of God we can all coexist. Introverts and extroverts and

everything in between.

God spoke clearly; Nissi was not the problem, but the world's perception of Nissi. God said, "This is a privilege!" My whole focus changed. From, "I HAVE TO do this," to "I GET to have this child."

—Nancy— (Mother)

✝

15. MY LIFE AS A SERVICE DOG

For from him and through him and for him are all things. To him be the glory forever! Amen.
-Romans 11:36 (NIV)-

(By Trix-C)

My first experience as a therapy dog involved working with low-functioning autistic children. I wanted to help them, but the constant abrupt noises, and unrestrained, sometimes violent tics freaked me out when I was alone with the kids. I needed my handler with me all the time. Because of the intense interaction, I suffered canine PTSD and washed out.

The first time I met Nissi, my new Mamma, my heart raced like a drum. Confused and a little scared, I approached her. Even though the surroundings were new and unfamiliar, the moment I saw the smile on her face, it clicked – working time! She reached out her hand, and I put my head underneath it. This made her so happy. I moved closer, and she scratched my back and belly. It was then we both just knew – we were made for each other.

The first few months were pretty amazing as we got to know each other. All I had to do was walk up to her, and she would feed me. We had so much fun together!

Getting to meet new people was exciting for both of us. Even though it was fun and exciting, sometimes the fear from my PTSD still surfaced in new situations. But I pressed my body up to her wheelchair, and I felt better. I helped her, too. My presence relieved a lot of the pressure for her to act or present herself in a certain way. We were a team. I knew she would protect me. She made me feel safe and I made her feel safe, too.

The real fun began when Mamma Nissi taught me to jump over things. We started with one simple jump. She put a treat on a yellow plate on the floor on the other side of an obstacle. When she gave the command, "Go to place," I jumped over the obstacle. And just like that, one jump turned into two, three and so on.

Seeing my Mamma happy made me want to do it faster, better, more. I picked it up so quickly, Nissi' dad, Luis, couldn't build enough obstacles for us.

Mamma started posting videos on Facebook. Before long, the videos went viral through the dog-trainer community. We became famous among several agility dog trainers around the world.

One of the things we loved doing together, was swimming! Because I'm older, Mamma insisted I wear a lifejacket when I went in the water. Mamma's mom, Nancy, swears we were cut from the same cloth because we love all the same things. Eating, lying around, swimming and people!

Sometimes Mamma would say, "I swear Trix-C understands what I am thinking," which, of course, I could. You see, I was able to sense when Mamma was unhappy or sick or even mad. When she felt bad, I always let her know I was right there with her.

For example, she had problems with her left leg. It cramped and gave her fits of great physical pain. Many times, when she lay on the couch with her leg out, I covered her leg with my body and took a little nap on it. She felt better, and I knew I did a good job.

We got to the point where I went to church without a leash. I felt so comfortable there. I knew everyone, and everyone knew me. I was always near her. Even when I eventually retired at 13, Mamma still took me to church.

So how does a service dog retire? Usually someone adopts retirees as a pet. My story is a little unusual: I was not a normal service dog.

When it was time for me to retire (too many aches and pains), my original trainer took me in. This was great, because I was in love with her dog. We got acupuncture together, played, and slept all day.

Mamma started training another dog, but two months later, when I saw her, I felt like I never left. I climbed on her tiny lap, and she cried her eyes out. She needed me!

Mamma's new dog did not work out— too hyper. Mamma called him the Energizer Bunny. Although he became the number two dog in the country, Zorro just wasn't a good match for her. Mamma needed someone calm, like me. Even her dad didn't yell around me. I brought calm..

A PARADOX OF VICTORY

So, I went home with Mamma for a visit over Thanksgiving Break. You have never seen a family cry so much over a dog. And, in case you are wondering, dogs cry, too!

You see, to Mamma there's no one like me, and to me there's no one like her.

From that moment on, I stayed with Mamma, although I was still officially retired. I was glad to be back, but some parts of retirement were hard. Mamma left home without me, even though I wanted to go everywhere. But I had no cartilage in my bones, and had lost both bone mass and muscle mass. Old age stinks. And the older I got, the more it stunk.

I tried to hold on so long for Mamma. Yes, I was in pain. When I couldn't take it anymore, I had to let Mamma know I needed to go. Just go. I fell down, looked at Mamma and let her know: I'm done!

She was a fierce Mamma bear, but she couldn't bear the thought of losing me. When she finally understood how much pain I was in, she knew it was time. She had to let me go.

I know she misses me. I know she always will.

✝

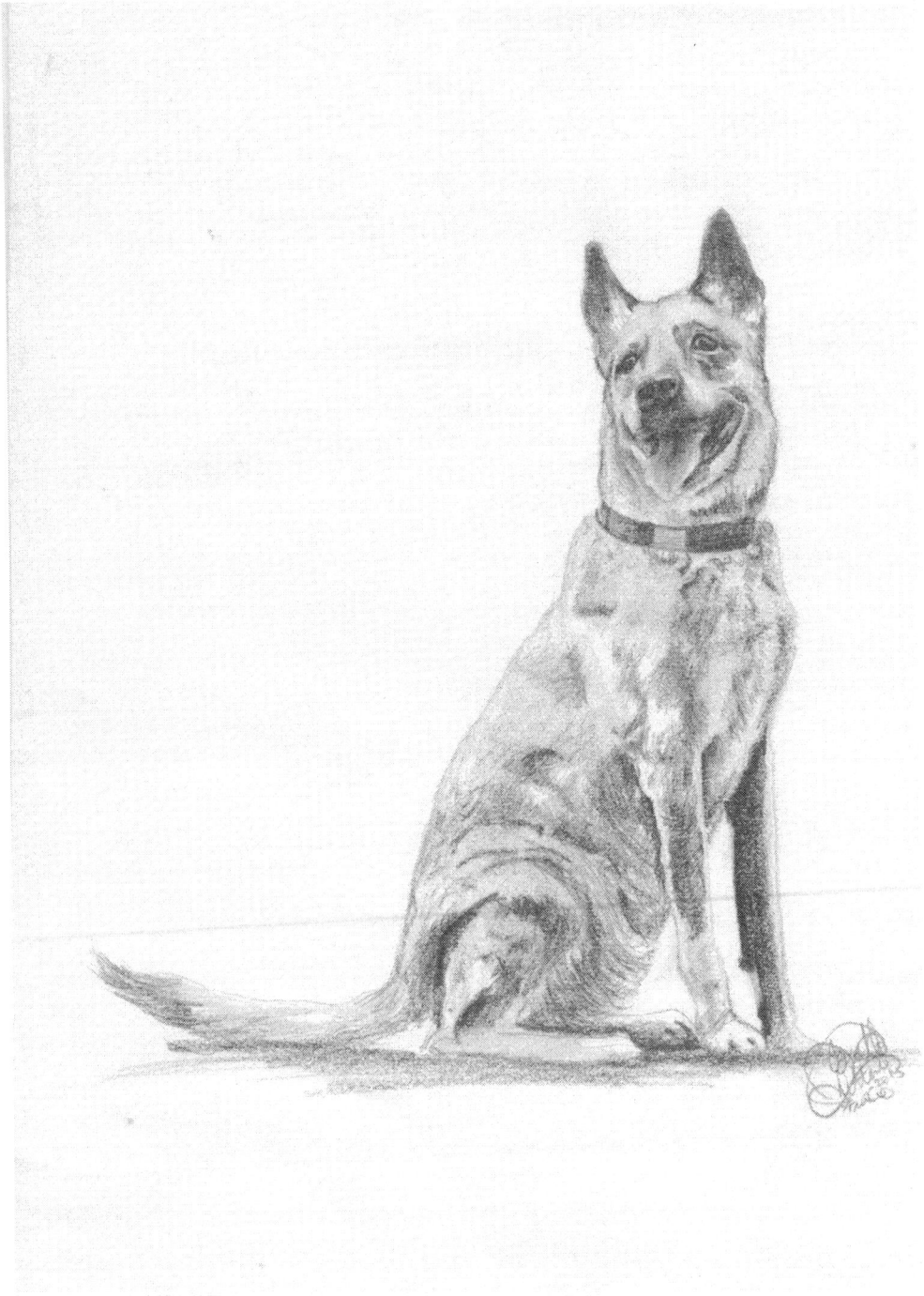

Nissi says:

That dog was worth all our cars combined – literally. She was a Belgian Malinois worth $75,000, unspayed. Of course, her value to us was way beyond money. She had my heart.

Ann, Tammy and I were training Apollo, a chocolate lab mix, but he turned out to be too dominant. The stress from training him brought on my first attack of shingles. Because Apollo was like... GOSH... Stress on steroids for me.

When Ann saw what was happening, she called my mom. "Let's try a little trick on Nissi. I will take Apollo for training, and Nissi can 'baby-sit' Trix-C for me. Then Nissi can see what a real service dog is like."

When Ann brought Trix-C for "baby-sitting", she simply said, "HERE'S your new dog," and handed me Trix-C's leash. That was it!

Tammy took Trix when she had to retire from service dog status. I am so thankful she had the selfless heart to recognize that Trix-C could never retire from being my dog. Because of Tammy, we got to spend Trix-C's final years together. I still get emotional when I think about that last year and a half with Trix-C. I will always treasure that time.

Trix-C made me realize I had to be strong for her because of her PTSD. I needed her, but she needed me, as well. Because of training with her, I learned how to present my confident self.

Some curious dogs are rude, and she corrected them. I would learn to recognize curiosity and take charge myself. Even with my severe disability, I learned to shield us from other dogs with just a look. I guess you could say we looked out for each other.

When Trix-C let me know she was dying, I just kept telling her, "You're killing me!" The pain was too much. I called my mom crying and crying. My sweet dog still tried to comfort me - even in her pain. She taught me it's OK to be a little scared.

At the end, we were both suffering. I couldn't bear the

thought of losing her, so it took a whole day for me to understand her pain was really too much. My mom took my beloved Trix-C to the doctor, who put an end to her suffering. Now, I suffer alone.

I miss her. I always will.

"Woof, woof, woof! Yip! Yip! Yip!"

—Gatsby—

WOOF!

—Luna—

"Dogs have a way of finding the people who need them, and filling the emptiness we didn't ever know we had"

—Thom Jones—

A PARADOX OF VICTORY

16. FEAR AND BEAUTY

"In riding a horse, we borrow freedom"

—Helen Thompson—

I happen to know someone who will go 150 mph on a motorcycle but won't get on a horse. That is so unfathomable to me. Why are you happy to risk your life on a piece of machinery balanced on just two wheels, but the thought of mounting a 1500 pound animal with four legs, terrifies you?

I have an actual reason to be scared of horses. When I was eight years old, we were looking for a family horse. My sister and I both had ridden horses for four years, so we wanted a horse of our own. I had ridden Lightning before, but this time, things went haywire. Divine and I saddled up - me in the front, my sister holding on to me. As my parents steadied us, a stallion that was being dismounted from a trailer spooked Lightning, who bolted like a bat out of hell. With two little girls holding on for dear life.

The next thing I remember, my parents scooped up Divine from the dirt. Without my parents holding me in place, my body began to jerk around, and I ended up spooking Lightning again. I don't remember what happened next, but I landed on the ground, too. The horse stepped on my leg and broke it in two places. I had to wear a cast from my ankle to my hip, and the 4 ½ weeks I wore that miserable cast were probably the hardest weeks I've ever lived.

Have you ever had an itch and haven't been able to scratch it? It's annoying, right? Now, imagine that times a million.

Instead of an itch, imagine it being excruciating pain.

That's the way it was for me. Not necessarily due to my broken leg, but because my leg was immobilized. Every time I had a spasm, the pain took over my body, and I cried and screamed from the torture of not being able to move. I don't think my mom and I slept for more than four hours a night during those 4 ½ weeks.

It took me over a year to get back on a horse and many years after that to trust horses again. But even while I didn't trust them, I still loved the feeling every time I rode! When you ride bareback, you feel every movement as though it is your own. This exhilarated me. So, I continued to ride until I was about nineteen.

Before my fall, I was fearless when it came to horses. The mental and physical journey to get back on a horse was long and hard. Sometime, between the first time I rode after my accident and the last time I got on a horse, I lost that fear.

Except for Lightning, the only experiences I had with horses were at the therapeutic horse-riding facility. So,

I really didn't know what normal horses were like. I can't just get on any old horse. It has to be trained for people with disabilities. Also, it has to be special. Where do you go to find a special horse? For me, it was the Satellite Center.

The Satellite Center employed trained professionals who taught basic riding skills. With side-walkers and someone leading the horse, my skill and confidence grew. Therapeutic horseback riding is probably one of the main reasons why I have such good balance. When you ride a horse, you have to have good balance, or you'll fall right off!

My family and I drove thirty minutes every week to get me on a horse to exercise my body. For seventeen years, it was the highlight of my week. At nineteen, I had to stop, because the drive was too much for my mom.

About a year after I had stopped riding at the Satellite Center, I went to a stable in my area. It was great, and further built my confidence in riding! I didn't really have a choice in the matter. The woman in charge told me, "You have perfect balance." So, she just put me on a horse and said, "Go!"

I loved it!!! But she didn't have a proper facility to accommodate my needs, so I ended up having to quit that as well. After that, I tried to get back into horses, but it was never the right time. Dog training became a big priority, and I felt like I didn't have any time left for horses. My health or my family's health - something always got in the away. So, with great regret, my riding days came to an end. I miss them still.

When I'm around livestock or any kind of farm or ranch, my heart cries out for the days I spent riding. Downtown San Antonio has always had horse carriage rides, and some of the drivers are sweet enough to let me hang out with the horses. But as much as I love spending time with them, there's really nothing like riding! Goodness, how I missed the feeling of riding astride a horse. I longed for that for the last 4 years.

My dreams finally came true. A few months ago, I met

Julie, a really cool girl at Physical Therapy. This beautiful ray of sunshine is a true cowgirl! She and her sister are part of a therapeutic horseback riding organization near my home called Hope Reins. They agreed to give me a lesson. To say I was excited would not be accurate. I was ecstatic!!!

According to my side walkers, Julie and her sister, I did pretty amazing for my first time back in the saddle. I owe it mostly to their beautiful mare, Beauty... and yes, that's her name! She seriously is the most gentle horse I've ever met. Even when I got wobbly, all she did was stop and wait patiently for me to recenter my body.

Driving home from that first ride, I was so happy I could cry. I felt like I was home again. Home to who I really was. Home to a familiar, overwhelming joy. I think she felt it, too. She responded so well to me. As a matter of fact, we will be competing in a showmanship competition where I guide her by her bridle and a leading rope in an arena.

The last time I felt this connected to an animal was with my precious service dog, Trix-C. Of course, no animal could ever hold a candle to her, but Beauty came pretty close!!!

Until one has loved an animal, a part of one's soul remains unawakened.

—Anatole France—

"A horse is the projection of peoples' dreams about themselves — strong, powerful, beautiful — and it has the capability of giving us escape from our mundane existence."

—Pam Brown—

"The essential joy of being with horses is that it brings us in contact with the rare elements of grace, beauty, spirit and freedom."

-Sharon Ralls Lemon-

17. MY CHEERLEADERS

Mentoring is a brain to pick, an ear to listen, and a push in the right direction.
—John C. Crosby—

Do you remember that one teacher? That teacher that reminded you of who you are as a person? A person with a purpose and destiny?

Well, I didn't have one of those.
I had about six.

Six wonderful mentors and teachers who supported me, stood up for me, taught me the value of life and what it means to be a woman of God. Some men also helped me

109

over the years, but today I want to focus on the women. The six women you will meet in this chapter believed in me when I didn't believe in myself. These women listened to my girly rants and shared wisdom in truth and love.

Luckily, I'm still close with most of them. In fact, one of them wrote the forward for this book! I'm also related to one. No, I'm not talking about my mom! She got her own chapter. She really deserves her own book. Really!

For their privacy, I will use only first names. Sharon, Wendy, Stephanie, Nancy (not Mom), Michelle and Nhora. Each one of these women bring their own unique beauty and wisdom to my life through the course of each friendship. Every single one, at one time or another, sat with me while I cried or threw a pity party. They have heard my frustrations and limitations first-hand. After each rant, they are quick to remind me who I am! They remind me of how far I've come and instill courage to continue forward in the struggles and restrictions of my life.

Sharon has been my mentor since high school. The woman is one of the most spiritual people I have ever known! She is so in tune with the Lord, it's scary! She can also read this girl like a book. With just a glance, she can tell if I am frustrated, angry or just hormonal. I survived some of the worst years of my life with her by my side encouraging me to fight back against depression and anxiety. I've known her for so long, that her son calls me his big sister, and I call him my little brother. Sharon helped me realize my full potential in God and as a woman! Even though our time together is limited, she continues to be an impactful presence in my life. So much so, that I asked her to write the foreword for this book. Thank you, Mama Green!

I've known Sweet Wendy since high school. She was one of the only leaders at youth group who would and could pick me up physically. Wendy has a very beautiful way of being able to speak love but also conviction with a soft voice. She's a native Floridian so we got along great: I'm a "go with the flow" kind of gal, and so was she. Even though she was actually more Bella's mentor, I don't think she'll ever know how much her gentle spirit spoke to me. She taught me you don't have to be physically strong to have a strong spirit. I don't get to see her often, but every time I do, I want to cry and tell her everything that's going on, because she would be so proud of me. She knew me when I felt like I was nothing, and she wanted to help me, and she did. Thank you, sweet Wendy!

Stefanie has been my mentor since I was at least 20. Stefanie is probably one of the sweetest humans I have ever known. And she is one of the most spiritual people I have ever known. It doesn't matter what I tell her, she never stops loving me, never stops meeting with me. Stefanie knows my deepest and darkest secrets. Stuff I would never tell my sister or even my best friend. She has seen me grow into the person I am today through a lens of anticipation. She often reminds me that she knew exactly who I was going to be. Not in a condescending way, but as a person who believed in me and saw me as my true self. Last time we met, she told me, "You're not done Nissi! There is so much more for you and you have only begun to scratch the surface." When she says something like this, it makes me want to both jump for joy and cry in a corner. She very gently reminds me I was never meant to be who I am by myself. Thank you, my darling Stefanie!

Nancy is one of my true cheerleaders! Mother to one of my best friends, she kinda adopted me into her family. I didn't have much choice in the matter. She said, "You're my new daughter!" She's as sassy as they come, which pretty much makes us soul sisters! She's never seen me as the girl in the wheelchair. And she would CUT anyone who would ever lay a finger on me! Being adopted into the family has made her as protective of me as she is for her own children. If she sees that I'm trying to accomplish something, she's one of the first to offer praise and encouragement. This caring woman never says anything she doesn't mean, which in my eyes is the biggest comfort. Lord knows I get plenty of praise from people who are trying to go the extra mile for the girl in the wheelchair. She doesn't see it that way, and I love that about her.

Thank you, Nancy.

The fierce Michele! I've known this woman since I was 12 years old. Her daughter became my sister's best friend. Don't get me wrong, I love her daughter, Jen! Truly! But anytime we went over, I'd love hanging out with Mama Michele. Jen and I were going to the same homeschool co-op, and sometimes the other mothers would whisper about me, because I wasn't as advanced as the other kids. Michelle was one of the first to stand up for me besides my mother. She was one of the truest Mama bears! Honestly, I have never had anyone that wasn't related to me stand up for me the way she did. I am truly grateful for the conversations we had and continue to have. Her love for Jesus and her amazing Alabama sass are always fun and exciting to be around. Thank you, Michelle for being in my corner when I needed you the most!

To the woman who is literally the fire beneath my butt! No one would dare talk to me the way my sweet Tia Nhora does! And I mean no one! Not even my own mother. My dear Tia Nhora has known me my whole life. But we truly become close over the last 15 years or so. She took care of me when I was in high school for a little bit. And after that, every so often, she would take me out to the movies, or we would just sit in the parking lot and eat pizza. For years, she was my date for Valentine's Day or if I just need to get away from it all. If I ever wanted to go to rally or a concert and my mother wouldn't take me, my Tia Nhora would be the first one to say, "Yes, let's go!"

But, like I said before, she was also the pain in my booty. She poked, prodded, and pushed and pushed and pushed until I actually did something with my life! I love her so much it hurts! Back when I was in high school, I used to call everybody "dude". So, she started calling me "dude", and it drove me bonkers. Now it's our call sign!

She loves being able to see my true potential! She highly encouraged (annoyed) me to get a service dog and I did. She's always encouraging me to do more, more, more! As my birthday present one year, she paid my way to do the Tough Mudder. On the other hand, she is the FIRST to let me know if I'm doing something I'm NOT supposed to be doing. Thank you for being a pain in my booty, Tia Nhora.

So, to my cheerleaders I want to say thank you for continually loving and supporting me. For believing I can be more, do more. For never doubting my abilities, in spite of my disabilities. I love you all dearly!

Go therefore and make disciples of all the nations, baptizing them in the name of the Father and of the Son and of the Holy Spirit, teaching them to observe all things that I have commanded you; and lo, I am with you always, even to the end of the age." Amen.
—Matthew 28:19-20-

18. JOHN H

A mentor is someone who sees more talent and ability within you, than you see in yourself, and helps bring it out of you.

-Bob Proctor-

From the time I was twelve to fourteen years old, I wanted to disappear from the world. I watched my sister, Bella, my identical twin, blossom from a tomboy into a girl with curves in the right places. I felt maybe God put me on the earth just as a contrast to showcase Bella's beauty - Beauty and the Beast of Pity. It didn't matter how many times my parents told me I was pretty, I saw the looks of others. They said to Bella, "Oh, you are so beautiful!" And, as an afterthought, to me, "You're pretty, too." Like I would believe that!

When people said to my mom, "You poor thing," or "I don't

know how you do it," or "Good job," my teenage brain interpreted it as, "What a burden your daughter is."

I felt like a scene in a movie where the focus blurs out everyone around me. No one understood me, and I didn't feel like they could comprehend or even care to know what was going on in my head. How could they understand it all anyway? I didn't even understand it myself.

So, I turned to God. Not on my knees, but with a fist raised in the air, shouting, "WHY? Am I here for the punch line for a very sick joke? To make my family look good, while I'm stuck in this stupid chair?"

I became very good at putting on a mask for people. In the back of my mind, I knew I was supposed to be a light in the world, even if I hated myself. Even though I was so angry at the one I was representing. But, at the pinnacle of my self-pity rampage, I met a very special person.

My parents decided it was time to change churches when I was fourteen. I hated it. I didn't want to change churches or anything else in my life. The only reason I went to Riverside Community Church in Bulverde, Texas, was because my mom said I could go to the middle school group. I was on the precipice of high school, but I didn't want to grow up.

As my mom pushed me toward the middle school area, two tables blocked the way. As we got closer, the man standing behind the tables smiled. "Can I help you?"

Mom said, "We were looking for the middle school group."

"We're just over here," he said moving the tables aside. Then, casually, as if he had known me his whole life, said, "I'll take her." He didn't think twice, even though he had never helped anyone with a disability before.

My world stopped at that moment, a million thoughts going through my brain, the loudest yelling, *What the heck is going on???* I had never experienced this kind of carefreeness toward me. The Lord flooded my heart with his mercy and love. I dumped the crappy attitude, started coming back to life!

He saw me - he didn't just see my chair. He wasn't

bothered by my circumstances. He made me feel normal. Immediately he took me under his wing. Without saying a word, he knew I needed someone who would stand up for me. Not only that, he knew what I wanted as a young teenager. He could look at me and picture the world through my eyes. And he reminded me constantly, "This is not impossible, Nissi".

The next few years with John as my youth pastor would probably be some of the best years of my life. He encouraged me to embrace my sassiness and to show people I could be more than just the girl in the wheelchair. He could see past the bullshit and see maturity. On many occasions, when I let boy-craziness take over in my high-school years, he would say, "I know you're better than that Nissi".

John made sure I never felt like an inconvenience or bother. For example: It was time for people to sign up for the mission trip to New Orleans, Louisiana. Bella felt like she wanted to go. Secretly I felt the same way. My parents decided to take us both to the first mission trip meeting. They told me not to get my hopes up, just in case. When we arrived at the meeting, John was so excited and insisted I go. I was so happy I could cry! It was on that mission trip I started realizing my calling in life - PEOPLE. It was also on that mission trip I met one of my best friends. (You'll meet Ben in the next chapter.)

On our way to New Orleans, we stopped at Sonic. As usual, I was the last one to finish eating. Which meant it was just me and John hanging out at the picnic tables. He took this time to inform me of something. "Nissi, I never want you to feel unincluded in whatever we do. Where there's a will, there's a way".

For the first time in my life, I felt like I had actual options. I didn't feel stuck anymore. I had liberty to choose! For years John encouraged me to share my story, and for years I fought it. So many times, our conversations consisted of me telling him how bored I was, and him saying, "Well aren't you going to do something about that? Nissi, you have a story to tell. Go out and tell it." Well, John Hinkebein, I'm telling it now!

✝

I get mad at her if she settles. "Get off your butt and do something. Dream more. push harder."
—John H- (Pastor)

✝

19. BENJAMIN

We've been friends for over 10 years. It was good for us get to know each other in a small group of people. There is only one other person I still talk to from high school... On the mission trip, carrying her up thirty stairs to where we were staying was easier than carrying the wheelchair. That was harder, and I could give that job to someone else.

—Ben— (Close friend)

I met Benjamin at our first mission trip meeting when I was 15 years old. Here's this string bean, super-white guy, wearing a burnt-orange jersey. His skinny legs dangled from his stool in front of the fireplace at the Loft Coffee House. Little did I know, he would impact my life in more ways than I could ever write down.

In his words: "We didn't have a choice but to become friends."

It's completely true! In spite of the fact that he is engineer-brained and plays sports (he is the only reason why I have the ESPN app on my phone), he had no choice but to spend time with me as we were squished in a van for HOURS!

Along with a few other guys on the mission trip, Ben had to carry me up and down a flight of stairs for about a week. So, I had to learn to trust him. That was a lot for someone like me, who did not trust easily. Especially when it meant I had to feel vulnerable.

But, it became easy to trust Ben. He made me feel safe. He never once saw me as "poor Nissi" in a wheelchair - EVER! Even though he was a quiet guy, he would manage to say things like, "Why do you eat so much? Lay off the pizza and the burgers! Some people have to actually pick you up and carry you around!" What a punk!

The boy was crazy! He deliberately rolled me into doorways and left me in hallways at stores. Even glaring looks from indignant shoppers didn't stop him. From that first summer, he made sure I felt like one of the gang. He, Bella and I went out with friends weekly, going to the movies and hanging out at the Loft Coffee House on Saturday nights.

The following year, we went on another mission trip. Because Ben was a senior in high school, I was afraid to lose him after he graduated. But amongst all the craziness of the mission trip, he made a promise to me: "I'll never abandon you. You can always come to me. No matter how far apart we are, we will always be friends." Those are powerful words, but even as an 18-year-old kid, he meant them.

Even when we were teenagers, he was a rock. Solid and there for me. But after he came back from being away at college for about 4 1/2 years, we truly became close friends. When Bella moved to Dallas, it was like an unspoken understanding between her and Ben, *Take care of my sister.* And he did. Even though I pestered the fire out of him, there was no one else our age around. So he was stuck with me.

The growth of our friendship went something like this:

(Texting)

Nissi: Wanna go to the movies?

Ben: Sure, I'll pick you up at 6.

Nissi: (an hour later): I'm broke. Gotta cancel.

Ben: No. Be ready when I get there.

Nissi: PHTTTT!!!! You're not the boss of me.

Ben: Yes, I am.

When one of my disabled friends passed away, I texted Ben to come to the funeral with me. I hate funerals (death and I don't get along so well), but I knew I had to be there. I wanted to go with Ben, because he lets me be myself. But, we encountered a problem: The stinker didn't tell me he had never been to a funeral before.

For some reason, he wheeled me down middle of the chapel, as close to the front as possible, right behind the family. Not an inconspicuous place. That's where the argument began in very loud whispers:

"I'm gonna take you out of your chair."

"Why?"

"Cause the coffin has to come down the middle aisle, right?"

"It's not a wedding, Ben."

We were trying to argue quietly: A tall guy. A girl with purple hair in a wheelchair. Front and center at a funeral. Who knew it was going to get worse. Much worse.

Ben insisted on clearing the aisle, so he hoisted me out of the wheelchair to put me on the pew. But, when he tried to bend my leg underneath me, he forgot to hold me up. Kerplop! I fell sideways. BAM! The sound of my bones hitting the hard-wooden bench echoed in the rafters.

A collective gasp sucked in all the air in the chapel. Everyone must have thought he was trying to kill me. A million well-meaning hands helped me upright. A million scolding glares aimed at Ben. When all was right, and everyone was seated, Ben leaned over and whispered, "Everyone is so touchy!"

I had to fight laughing my way through the funeral.

Nonchalant is kind of Ben's default setting. Sometimes, I wonder if Ben has that Bob Marley song playing in his head:

"Don't worry about a thing
'Cause every little thing gonna be alright..."

Like, sometimes my seat belt gets stuck in the frame of my manual chair. It's impossible to get the buckle out if I'm sitting in it. Instead of being frustrated, he just lifts me out of the chair (which he just assembled), fixes the seatbelt, and plops me right back down, all secure. Not complaining once. Lots of other people get frustrated in this situation - especially in the blistering heat of South Texas. Or when it's raining. But not Ben. Not once. Not ever.

The dork has something against ramps. For as long as I can remember, he insists on bumping me down a flight of stairs rather than a ramp. I think he does it because he knows I'm secretly an adrenaline junkie. He humors me, you know.

One of my very wise older friends describes Ben as someone who will never make a decision without thinking about it first. Ten years we've been friends, and I've yet to see him mad. No joke! It's like he's missing a wire or something.

He'll go extra fast in his Camaro. He knows how much I love the feeling of going fast. It's kind of our thing. Not to mention, NOBODY else would ever do that with me in the car or take the risks he takes going downstairs. While everyone is trying to protect me, Ben lets me fly!

Benjamin makes me feel invincible in certain aspects of my life! When I told him I wanted to do the Tough Mudder, he didn't question my decision like most people. He simply said: "You'd better train!"

A few years ago, my best friend met the woman of his dreams. Within a year, they were married. I'm not going to lie, I thought I was gonna lose my best friend forever. But Karen graciously puts up with all my craziness. She has beautifully accepted me, and, on one occasion, even had to assist me in the restroom. She didn't flinch. Pretty incredible!

Ben is one of three people in my life, besides my family, who I would trust with anything. My parents would trust him with me full-heartedly. Ten years ago, if you would've asked me, "Do you think you guys are gonna be around in 10 years?"

My answer would've been, "No."

I'm a little neurotic and Ben is stoic. But, now I wouldn't have it any other way. In the friend department, Ben is top three! Ok, top two. But don't tell him.

Give, and it will be given to you. A good measure, pressed down, shaken together and running over, will be poured into your lap. For with the measure you use, it will be measured to you.

-Luke 6:38 (NIV)-

20. ALEXANDER

One of the most beautiful qualities of true friendship is to understand and to be understood.

-Lucius Annaeus Seneca -

Have you ever met someone, and right off the bat you knew were going to be good friends?

That's the way it was when I met Alex. When Bella was sixteen, she went to music camp and came back interested in a boy. A few months later, when I finally met him, I could see why Bella liked him: His sweet smile and gorgeous blue eyes drew me in. I felt safe around him.

I can honestly say, I don't think I've laughed with anyone else as much I have with Alexander. Although his

133

relationship with Bella was long-distance, he visited regularly. On those frequent visits, Alex got to see the good, the bad and the ugly of Nissi Salazar. I remind him all the time that he's one of the few people that can get me from calm-as-a-cucumber to the Incredible Hulk in a matter of seconds. A true brother.

The first time he fed me, we were waiting for Bella to get off work. Since we were both hungry, he bought pizza. When it arrived, we kind of just stared at each other for what seem like a full minute. I was waiting for him to feed me. He was waiting for me to tell him how to feed me.

We both burst out laughing and, just like that, he became one of the few people to automatically take initiative to feed me. That means a lot to a girl who is always hungry. And so much more. Not only does he load me in and out of cars, and push me here, there, and everywhere, but he always encourages me to do whatever my heart desires. He is one of the few people I trust completely.

You can imagine how I felt when Alex and Bella broke up. But, despite his break up with my sister, my friendship with Alex grew over the years. Although he is a brilliant engineer, most of the time we talk about stupid, meaningless stuff. But our friendship is so meaningful. While Ben brings out my adventurous side, Alex makes me feel like a kid again. He brings out a wild and crazy part of me that is just so much fun! I need fun in my life.

Amongst all the laughter, being with him reminds me just how wise and thoughtful he is. He can read me like a book. He can discern a look or a tone in my voice and say, "What are you really thinking, Nissi?" Even though he might already know, he wants me to say it aloud.

When he was ready to propose to his girlfriend, he was worried about if I would be a little neurotic about one of my best friends getting married. "Don't worry, Nissi. You are always going to be in my life." And, true to his word, he still checks in whenever he can.

The day I turned 21, I was blessed to have the flu. *NOT!!* Even though I was running a fever and heavily medicated, I was determined to celebrate with the twin and my family. Since Alex and my brother were in town, we decided to go to brunch at The Cheesecake Factory. I was so excited to order my first alcoholic beverage. Bella ordered her drink.

Then it was my turn: "I'll have an OSMOSIS, please."

The waitress hesitated for a moment. "An OSMOSIS?..." She looked a little confused.

"Yeah... you know... that tropical drink with a little umbrella..."

Before I could finish my sentence, Alex and my brother, Stephen, burst out laughing. Through chuckles, Alex choked out, "I think she wants a MIMOSA!"

To this day, Alexander still teases me about it. Our conversations usually go something like this:

Nissi: That's funny!

Alex: You know what's really funny?

Nissi: What?

Alex: The time you ordered an osmosis!!

Nissi: ALEXANDER!!!

Alex: Hahahahahaha!!!!

Recently, I had a discussion with Alex about this very chapter in my book. I asked him, "What do you want the world to know about me?"

Without missing a beat, he said, "I want people to know that you have never complained about your situation. That even when you're in pain, you were always looking at the bright side of things. Oh, and don't forget to tell them you're extremely weird."

Ladies and gentlemen, my best friend Alejandro!!

Here's what I want the world to know about Alex:
Alex is the person who gets me out of my head in a crisis.

✝

He has helped me get through some really tough times, bringing me out of the dumps with his stupid jokes. They are the kind of jokes that are so bad, they're good.

And he is really good at bad jokes!

It is one of the blessings of old friends that you can afford to be stupid with them.

-Ralph Waldo Emerson-

21. MACIE

Many people will walk in and out of your life, but only true friends will leave footprints in your heart.

-Eleanor Roosevelt-

Macie was an annoying 13-year old. The first time I met her, she was a tall lanky preteen who didn't know her own body. For a "mature" 15-year old girl like me, two years was like a lifetime between us. Seeing "children" like her giggle about boys made me cringe. Besides, Macie came from a wealthy family, and I lived in a different world.

I vowed never to become friends with someone younger than me. Because of the unique challenges of my life, I always felt so much older than people my age. My circle included adults. Two of my best friends were older than me, and both were guys. Secretly, I prayed for a close girl-friend for years, but for some reason, I never really got along with girls. Nothing against my own gender. It's just that it was always easier for me to talk to guys.

But the Lord doesn't operate according to our comfort. Instead he'll bring the most unlikely precious humans to our lives!

Looking back, I wish I could say we've been close for all those years. When people see us together, laughing and having a good time, most think we have been friends forever. The truth of the matter is, I've only really **known** her for about two years. Everything changed when I had a real conversation with Macie. No longer would I ever see her as loud and insincere. God answered my prayers with an unexpected friendship, and, wow, has it been fun!!

My best friend is strong (physically and emotionally). She played volleyball in high school and college. Standing at 5 feet, 10 inches, she's a beast. On many occasions I've called her my bodyguard. Mace has had heartbreak, betrayal, loss and grief just like everyone else. But she doesn't let it really get to her. In the midst of all these things, she continues to be joyful, funny, wise beyond her years, and one of the most compassionate people I have ever known.

But, I can't take her anywhere: She's beautiful, and all the boys want her! Like me, she has emotional and physical scars and, like me, she's learning to overcome them. But her scars are wrapped in a beautiful, blonde, legs-for-days package!

I had the most amazing opportunity to have my sweet best friend be my paid attendant for about a year-and-a-half. Having your best friend as your employee presents challenges in both work and relationship. Sometimes the lines blurred between friendship and work.

We had to learn how to set boundaries. We had to learn the rhythm of "workdays" vs. "hang-out days". Because of the working nature of our circumstances, Macie had to give, give, give to the point where, some days, she felt like my own personal punching bag. She wasn't just there for emotional friendship needs, she had to take care of the constant physical demands that my disability requires. Unfortunately, I took advantage of that. But because of our deep love for each other, we worked through those road bumps and our friendship deepened.

Our neediness for each other is actually more of a grounding. Sometimes, we just have to have a good cry and a hug. Not a talk, necessarily, just a cry and hug. It's like our brains and our hearts are connected so deeply that we NEED to touch.

One of the most beautiful things about our friendship is that we both want to be authentic. It's our driving force and our common ground. We've learned to remind each other, "You are not a people-pleaser. Don't be a people-pleaser." Of course, we say this because we are. But we are on a journey together to become comfortable with who God has made each of us to be.

Who would have thunk that annoying, middle-schooler would have become a gorgeous, wise, discerning woman who helps me find my center.

And who would have thunk that "mature" me could help her learn that imperfection has a beauty all its own.

Who says God doesn't have a sense of humor. Even though we come from opposite worlds, we not only have a **functioning** relationship, we have an **epic** friendship. From the outside, there's no explanation for us, which is why it makes perfect sense to me.

I love my Boo!

You did not choose me, but I chose you and appointed you so that you might go and bear fruit—fruit that will last—and so that whatever you ask in my name the Father will give you.

—John 15:16 (NIV)—

22. MY OWN PERSONAL DAYCARE CENTER

"Remember that mentor leadership is all about serving. Jesus said, 'For even the Son of Man came not to be served but to serve others and to give his life as a ransom for many.'"
—Tony Dungy

Ninety percent of the book you're reading was edited at one place, a coffee house near my home in Bulverde, Texas. The Loft is no ordinary coffee house. Not only do they serve great coffee, smoothies, and food - it's also a place of love, hope, inner healing and so much more. For me, it's my home away from home. It's where I go when it's too hard to just be stuck at home.

At first, I went to meet my mentor twice a month. Because

the coffee shop is a ministry of my church, I run into a lot of people I know. But a lot of other people hang out there. A lot of people. Every week, I look forward to a whole morning meeting new people.

I started out just meeting a friend there every couple of weeks, but as I went more often, the staff stepped in to help me. A few of the employees and volunteers actually began to take their break time to feed and talk with me. Now, three-and-a-half years later, I spend every Tuesday morning there, and 80% of the staff knows me and helps me.

A year after continually hanging out there, I realized they only charge me half-price for everything I even have my own button on the register now. It's so great! I still have a hard time believing they do this for me. Even now, it brings tears to my eyes. I come from a family that lives from paycheck to paycheck, and this gift The Loft gives me means the world to me and my family.

Because of The Loft, I am able to engage people from all

walks of life. Some of the best discussions I've had, and wisdom I've heard, has been at this little coffee house in Bulverde, Texas. It truly is my own personal daycare center! A place where I feel safe, loved and welcomed. Besides all that, it's the best cafe north of San Antonio!

For more information about:

Riverside Community Church visit:

connect2riverside.com

The Loft Coffee House visit:

theloftcoffeehouse.com

If I speak with human eloquence and angelic ecstasy but don't love, I'm nothing but the creaking of a rusty gate. If I speak God's Word with power, revealing all his mysteries and making everything plain as day, and if I have faith that says to a mountain, "Jump," and it jumps, but I don't love, I'm nothing. If I give everything I own to the poor and even go to the stake to be burned as a martyr, but I don't love, I've gotten nowhere. So, no matter what I say, what I believe, and what I do, I'm bankrupt without love.

–1 Corinthians 13:1-4 MSG–

23. HOME AWAY FROM HOME

"It is not how much you do, but how much love you put in the doing."
—Mother Teresa—

Over the years, I've always required some sort of physical therapy. I've experienced everything from very non-traditional therapy centers to very traditional therapy centers. I've had good and bad experiences in both.

From the beginning, therapy was never about what I wanted, but what I needed to make me functional. Even as early as four-years-old, therapy meant being manipulated - poked and massaged, forced to crawl (sounds simple, but...no).

✝

As I got older, I began to realize how most of these things were good for me, but my rebel spirit still didn't wanna have anything to do with them. "Exercise" was an ugly word - until 16-years-old when I started going to a little clinic in my small town.

The first time I walked through the doors of Smithson Valley Physical Therapy, my skepticism probably showed on my face. I didn't expect this place to be any different from the other cringe-worthy PT experiences in my life. Even with the friendly, accepting atmosphere, it still took me a good month to feel comfortable - my trust issues continued to flare up. Until I met Aaron.

Aaron was the most soft-spoken human I have ever met. And I could tell he wanted to know me - not just my body, not only my disability, but the human inside. For several years as he worked on my scoliosis and other issues he took time to listen to me. Because of Aaron's gentleness and genuine concern, I learned to trust a physical therapist for the first time.

One of the best neuro physical therapists in San Antonio decided to plant herself in this small little clinic, and I became one of her biggest fans. Selena took literally broken people and made them feel whole and confident in themselves again. Before I met her, I didn't think I would ever be able to transfer myself on and off my chair or stand up with limited assistance. She gave me confidence to believe in myself. If there's a theme for this book, it is this: I am who I am today because the Lord has put people in my life to plant seeds. Selena planted the seed of wanting to be physically free.

Unfortunately, all good things must come to an end, and Selena decided to part ways with our little clinic. We all miss her even to this day, staff and patients alike. After she left, PT became more of an obligation. I kind of just glided through on autopilot. For a while, I was just going for the social aspect of the experience.

Then I met Roger. For the first time in MY LIFE I started feeling like I could actually be physically independent. When they initially paired me with Roger, everybody warned me he was the hardest PT Assistant. But I didn't believe them. BIGGEST mistake! After our first session, I was sore for a whole week afterwards. But I loved every moment of it. After that, I started requesting him. Despite his demanding therapies, I called him "Sweet Roger."

Like a crazy person, I actually looked forward to getting beat up twice a week. Roger never limited me. If I wanted to try something new, he always said, "Sure! Why not?!"

One of my favorite things to do with Roger is planting my feet. Which means is I'm laying down on the mat and he straightens my legs and ankles and plants them on his chest. Then he pushes against them. When he does this, it gives my body the illusion that I'm standing, and it causes my body to relax.

Roger is in ridiculous good shape. Seriously! So, when my feet are planted on his chest, I usually take the opportunity to tease him about how his chest is squishy. In fact, I'm not the only one who likes to tease him.

Aaron and his wife have prayed over their business for it

to have a family dynamic. I'm going to be honest, they're not paying me to say this or anything like that. They really are like a loving, encouraging family over there. And if you go there long enough, you become family! Everything about it screams the presence of God. There's nothing like it anywhere else.

"Too often we underestimate the power of a touch, a smile, a kind word, a listening ear, an honest compliment, or the smallest act of caring, all of which have the potential to turn a life around."

—Leo Buscaglia, author—

Speak up for those who cannot speak for themselves, for the rights of all who are destitute. Speak up and judge fairly; defend the rights of the poor and needy.

—Proverbs 31:8-9 NIV—

✝

24. TOUGH MUDDER

Rebellion and adventure look a lot alike unless you know her heart. Physical looks like rebellion—Spiritual looks like adventure. She welcomes a challenge because of her adventurous spirit.

-John H— (Pastor)

Another crazy family get-together, and I got squished between two of my older cousins at dinner: Jeffrey was to the left of me and Christina to the right. We enjoyed the usual chit-chat about how life was going etc., etc.

At that time, I was pretty much doing **nothing** with my life. To say I was bored, would be the biggest understatement of the world. I was going through life on autopilot. Not really going anywhere, not really doing anything: I ached for adventure!

✝

Jeffrey started talking about all the exciting things he saw at the Tough Mudder, a 13-mile obstacle course through mud and over walls. Even though he had run it at least six times, I had only heard about the course on social media and through Bella. She wanted to do one with a group of friends to see whether not it would be accessible for me.

A mud-soaked torture run for a girl in a wheelchair. Made sense to me.

The more Jeffrey explained how it worked, the more it got me thinking, because the sole purpose of the Tough Mudder Race is INCLUSION. Young and old, and pretty much if you can breathe, you're more than welcome. I saw a YouTube video of a guy with no legs and no arms running the race!

TEAMWORK is the other selling point. It's more like a religious statement! No man gets left behind! If you don't have a team, you never have to worry about getting over some of the obstacles - There's always someone willing to lend a hand.

And then, Jeffrey looked straight at me and said, "You know what Nissi? I think you can do the Half Tough Mudder."

You might find it hard to imagine that the idea of running the Tough Mudder, one of the most popular and challenging obstacle courses in the U.S., would appeal to a girl in a wheelchair. After all, able-bodied teams labor through it and find it extremely challenging, requiring months of training.

OF COURSE, I wanted to do it! My life is a virtual endurance course, why not accept the challenge of a **literal** endurance course.

But even before the actual race, obstacles started appearing like brick walls. From past experience, I understood how to differentiate truth from lies. And I knew from the bottom of my heart the obstacles popping up were just lies.

I went straight to my physical therapy assistant, showed him a video, and stated firmly. "I want to do that!"

Roger, not all that surprised, asked, "Are you sure?"

"Yes."

"OK, it's gonna be hard, but I will help, and we will get you as ready as possible."

The first few months, although brutal, were so much fun and eye-opening. I didn't realize before how strong I was. I began to discover my own potential for independence.

In addition, Robin Gray started me on a weekly yoga routine, and I started re-teaching myself how to crawl (a skill I lost from inactivity).

The doctor put me on an anti-fungal diet. For someone who HATES to diet, you can imagine my suffering. There were days where it was physically painful as my body flushed toxins. Some days, I couldn't hold anything down: years of unhealthy eating was trying to force its way out of my body.

I love food, but I hate food.

After I started my diet, and as people began to take an interest in my journey, motivation compelled me to stick to it. I cheated rarely in the five months leading to the race. I even impressed myself with my dedication! TO A DIET!!!

Even worse than the diet? HIVES! Recurring, itchy-as-hell, maddening hives!

Even worse than hives? SHINGLES! Stress-induced, bone-deep pain, that drilled into every nerve. The itching itself was unbearable, but the second I tried to scratch, just the touch turned into fire. It's the level of pain that people have surgery for. The fact that it was on my back, kept me from ever relaxing in my chair. So add muscle fatigue and nausea to the mix. Not that I have any enemies, but if I did, I wouldn't wish this on my worst enemy.

With open sores, infection was a serious (and I mean SERIOUS) problem. Up until two weeks before the race,

I had to consider the possibility that a virus might sideline me and all my plans.

Here's a partial list of my team of eighteen:

- **Adam,** the Spiderman of our group, who conquered each obstacle like a piece of cake
- **Ben Matthewson** carried me, as always...
- **Bella...** my voice!!
- **Peter,** my "go-to" person. Right there all the time. Got me in and out of the chair.
- **Victor Prieto,** cousin, raised right next door
- **Nhora Prieto,** Aunt, my "Lamaze coach" for the race
- **Jeffrey,** team captain, knew the course well
- **Maddie,** friend of Divine
- **Michael,** with a ginormous heart. Didn't even know him, but it felt like having a brother on the course with me. When I was so tired, he held me and kept me from getting trampled.
- **Michelle,** who said, "I don't know what I'm doing here, but here I am!"

- **Paige Holden,** BEAST!

- **Roger Moreno,** Tough Mudder Dad

- **Haley Moreno,** youngest team member, but boy was she able to keep up.

- **Carmen Moreno,** Roger's wife, who ran the race to support him and me

- **Andrew,** PT support and one of my fans!

- **Crystal,** part of the PT family

- **Sara,** more of the PT family

- **Julian,** a friend of Peter's, experienced competitor

Finally, after weeks of planning and training, the day arrived:

In the car with my cousins and sisters on the way to the race was the sweetest time ever. Just what I needed to calm down. They teased me about my MOANA soundtrack as I sang along at the top of my little lungs.

Of course, we got lost. Really lost. Victor gave the GPS the wrong address. He never gets things wrong, so we were all laughing. As a result, we arrived late. Really,

really late: Got there like five seconds before the start. No time to think.

For a split second, at the starting line, I thought, *I can just go home*. I named my sister as the one to shoo off all the "mommies" - two in the race, three more in the cheering section. Knowing I had to concentrate, I told Bella, "Just keep them away from me. Especially anyone who is not 100% positive. I just can't handle it.

By the time we got in position, I was in the right mindset: I couldn't control anything! Before that moment, it was all about **me**. Now it was about **US** – this team of strong, willing, fearless people who loved me enough to put themselves through hell for the next few hours. We were focused and ready!

I didn't know what was going on at each part of the race. I didn't know anything. Now was the time to put my trust in my friends who were about to fully immerse themselves into helping me achieve an absolutely impossible task - Tough Mudder (Half), which the website describes as "five miles of mud and obstacles specifically designed to test your teamwork and toughness...you'll overcome mud-drenched obstacles and adrenaline-pumping challenges."

As pumped as I was, my team exceeded my energy. Terror!!! Excitement! Adrenaline pumping like no one's business! "Overwhelmed" doesn't even begin to describe the numbing emotions racing through my brain.

Yeah, we were crazy, but I said, "Let's do this! Just don't ask me anything, because I don't have any idea what I am doing!" I don't remember if the race started with a gunshot. I just remember, the next thing I knew, we were off!

First obstacle - BARBWIRE. My mom broke into tears. She thought I was suffering. Helpless, she ran to the next obstacle and waited for two hours, praying. That was her version, but the truth is Momma Bear got lost (I guess it runs in the family), so she just sat down and prayed. She said that God led her there.

And, boy, did we need prayer! Facing obstacles with names

like Kiss of Mud, Hold Your Wood, and Six Feet Under, I'm glad Momma prayed us through.

Besides crawling, dragging, climbing and hoisting, at one point, my team members strapped me on a log and carried me through the designated obstacle. That was my favorite part of the whole race.

Near the end, when everyone was good and exhausted, my wheelchair gave out. It broke and refused to cooperate. Lucky Ben got to carry me the rest of the way. Never complained, just carried me. Kinda like that song, "She ain't heavy, she's my sister...."

Throughout the race, my team kept me hydrated with water and bananas. They were especially diligent with the bananas. If I didn't have a banana in my mouth, someone was shoving one in. Of course, everyone kept asking if I needed to go to the bathroom. Of course, I lied.

Inevitably, toxins built up in my body. At the last obstacle, I collapsed against Bella, "I need water. Please get everyone away..." Even though she was exhausted, too, my little mother-hen twin became bodyguard and comforter. Nurse and refuge.

At the end of the race, my body went into shock. A dozen people bombarded me with cameras and congratulations, but all I could manage to think and say was, "Get this harness off me now!"

Ben Toalson, filming for the documentary he was making about me and the race, came back with the camera. "One last shot," he said. "Don't hit me!"

He's really lucky I was so exhausted, or his nose would have been toast.

I went limp in Roger's arms. He, Bella and Aunt Nhora started peeling off the outer layer of my wet clothes as I shivered from exhaustion. Even with temperature in the 90's, I was cold and delusional.

The hardest part?

Delegating, speaking, communicating, planning. Education without a curriculum. Through love and encouragement, I

had to connect, speak, communicate. Body, spirit, and mind all engaged. Mom said it was like a college education for me.

The easiest part?

Don't know if it was easy: But, oh, the feeling at the finish line! Nothing like it! In those five long hours of sweat, mud, tears and pain, I learned so much about myself, my friends, and my family.

But it was all worth it. The hard parts, the challenging parts, the trust built by my teammates. The Tough Mudder provided a way for people to see me how my life operates - not just obstacles, but that I needed a team, just like in my life. We are never meant to be alone.

The race gave me vivid pictures of how pure will can get me to a lot of places. I can try anything. Doesn't matter if it seems impossible. The race magnified my control issues, but putting me in the most challenging event of my life and stripping me completely of control. In surrendering control, I learned I have amazing friends and the most incredible family.

Scripture teaches when you love your neighbor as yourself you experience "shamah", the glory of God. By helping me, God gave them an opportunity to experience that. That is why I am here...

Six months into training, my friend Joanna Franco met me for coffee. When I told her what I was planning, the idea for the documentary, TOUGH NISSI, was born. In Joanna's words:

"This is the story about someone who thought she could not do the impossible, but yet achieved greatness.

"I was looking for a project, and as Nissi was preparing for the race, I said, 'This story needs to be told. Is there any way we can make this a documentary?'

"We both got super excited She became part of my process. Then Ben Toalson jumped in with both feet as videographer. He gave 200 percent in the planning, filming, scoring and editing.

"Before we knew it, the project exploded into an event, and Tough Nissi premiered December of 2017 to receptive audiences."

To learn more about TOUGH NISSI: toughnissi.com

If she was gonna do this there is no way I was gonna miss it. My job (along with Bella) was to make sure Nissi's voice and opinions were honored in the race.

—Ben— (Close friend)

But those who wait for the LORD's help find renewed strength; they rise up as if they had eagles' wings, they run without growing weary, they walk without getting tired.
—Isaiah 40:31 NET—

"Fear and selfishness are commonly known today as 'survival of the fittest, or 'the drive to survive', or 'kill or be killed,' or 'watch out for me first'. It is the polar opposite of giving, love or beneficence, and is the infection that is destroying God's creation"
—T R Jennings—

"Do you see what this means—all these pioneers who blazed the way, all these veterans cheering us on? It means we'd better get on with it. Strip down, start running—and never quit! No extra spiritual fat, no parasitic sins. Keep your eyes on Jesus, who both began and finished this race we're in. Study how he did it. Because he never lost sight of where he was headed—that exhilarating finish in and with God—he could put up with anything along the way: Cross, shame, whatever. And now he's there, in the place of honor, right alongside God. When you find yourselves flagging in your faith, go over that story again, item by item, that long litany of hostility he plowed through. That will shoot adrenaline into your souls!"

—Hebrews 12:1-3 (MSG)—

25. YOSEMITE

I look up to the mountains;
does my strength come
from mountains?
No, my strength comes
from GOD, who made
heaven, and earth, and mountains.
Psalm 121:1-2

Tired, cold and hormonal! A very bad combination, and my sisters and mom were tired of my bad behavior. I only slept for about 45 minutes the night before we arrived in California. Not to mention, I almost fell out of bed many times in our hotel room.

You know that saying, "Don't bite the hand that feeds you." Well, I was chomping like a T-Rex!

My sister, Bella, very adamantly reminded me that she

✝

wanted to go climb the mountains. "Are you SURE that's OK with you?" she asked.

Like a dummy I kept saying, "Yeah. Sure. No problem," when clearly it was a big problem for me. I wanted to be selfish. I wanted to climb that mountain, too.

As many people know, I love a good challenge. But every so often, I have to admit my limitations. Admitting I couldn't accept the challenge of climbing El Capitan (which a week before had claimed the life of an experienced climber) made me shake with anger. And I let everyone know it. Repeatedly.

I'm a firm believer in having a positive attitude. Bad behavior is a choice. And I was making all the wrong choices on the road to Yosemite National Park.

Our first day in the valley, Bella said, "Let's try the wheelchair accessible trails first." I tried to have fun. Part of me did, but I still wanted to climb mountains.

By the second day, like any good sister or mother, they made sure I knew they were fed up with my attitude. Which infuriated me even more. I kept thinking, *I'm the chill one. Why do you say I am acting crazy!?!*

The second I asked myself that question, I knew the answer: Besides my hormones acting insane, it all came down to pure jealousy! Irrational jealousy.

Oh, and don't forget self-pity.

You see, this was Bella's dream, not mine. When that thought became clear, my self-pity started to subside, and the jealousy fell away.

When I realized I had to be content with just looking, I couldn't believe what I was seeing. It was in that instant I started to see the beauty and the true majesty of Yosemite. Words like "spectacular" and "wonderful" can't even begin to communicate how beautiful Yosemite is.

I was speechless! The grandeur of it made me realize how

tiny I am in this great big world. Oh, how I was missing out by complaining! But, oh, how I wanted to explore!

When you're down in The Yosemite National Park Valley, to the left you have Half Dome and to the right you have El Capitan. And don't forget The Three Brothers and Yosemite Falls and Glacier Point - I could go on and on. Vast, indescribably grandeur! You truly can't escape from the intensity of it all.

It smelled like fall, but not a heavy musky, just a hair of smokiness. The Valley made me feel like I was in a cathedral, and God just brought heaven to earth with a "BAM." It felt like the whole place was worshipping God. You want to experience in every way. It engages all of your senses. It's the kind of place that makes you want to wrap yourself in a blanket and eat soup.

A great man named John Muir is the reason why Yosemite is a national park today. This is what he believed:

"Everybody needs beauty as well as bread,

places to play in and pray in,
where nature may heal
and give strength to body and soul."

I'm inclined to agree with him!

After God gave me an attitude adjustment, my mom and I started having so much fun! I can't tell you how many times we got lost in the valley, laughing the whole time! I had many opportunities to talk with some incredible people.

As a matter fact, one of those amazing people challenged me to go to all 58 national parks! This woman had a fear of heights and, like a boss, she wanted to conquer her fears. So, she became a rock climber. My HERO! She also told me about a program about adaptive rock climbing suited for people like me.

Speaking of challenges and disabilities. Yosemite is one of the most accessible places I've ever been!!! Every door has a button and every sidewalk has a ramp. The buses taking people from trail to trail always accommodated me first!

175

I would encourage anyone who is disabled to go visit Yosemite Valley! Next time, I'm most definitely taking my power chair and leaving everybody in the dust.

Because I am disabled, I am allowed to go to ALL national parks for FREE. Anyone want to join me?

By the way, I probably won't be climbing all the mountains (maybe just a few!)

P. S. - Special thanks to my Mama Bear who pushed me up and down the valley, and who was my personal photographer. You can see the photos on my blog. (http://justmebynissi.blogspot.com)

Thank you to my Bella for putting this whole thing together and for encouraging us to be adventurous!

Thank you to Divine for just being Divine! Pun intended...

All of us (Mom, Nissi, Bella and me) are interesting when we are together, because we all think we are right - even when we are wrong. Sometimes we get moody. In the car on the way, I was moody every now and then, but Nissi was so moody - the whole way to Yellowstone. She was throwing tantrums every five seconds! We were all thinking, Nissi! Chill out! When we finally arrived, I was so happy that Bella wanted to go hiking, because usually everyone wants to just hang out and do nothing.

—Divine— (Sister)

The LORD is gracious and righteous;
Our God is full of compassion.
The LORD protects the simple-hearted;
When I was in great need, he saved me.
Be at rest once more, O my soul,
For the LORD has been good to you.
For you, O LORD, have delivered my soul
from death, my eyes from tears, My feet
from stumbling, That I may walk before the
LORD in the land of the living.
Psalm 116:5-9

26. CONCUSSION

"We are all faced with a series of great opportunities brilliantly disguised as impossible situations."

—Chuck Swindoll—

The easiest part about having a concussion is getting a concussion.

Two-o'clock in the morning, half awake, I reluctantly called out to my mom. Half asleep herself, she settled me on the ivory throne to do my business. A few minutes later, I told her I was done.

"OK," she yelled from the other room. Hearing footsteps, I assumed she was in front of me. With my eyes still closed, I leaned forward, thinking she was standing there to catch me.

She wasn't!

Instead of landing on Mom like I do every single day of my life, I became one with the floor, the tub, and the wall. The shock jolted me more than the actual impact. For several seconds, I tried to make my mind understand what just happened. When I finally realized, I began to laugh and cry at the same time. My mom sprang into action, feeling around my body making sure nothing was broken. Satisfied, she picked me up and carried me to bed.

"Mama...my head...my head." Without missing a beat, she placed an ice pack on my head. I fell asleep to my mom praying for me and woke up to her checking my head for bruises. My sweet mother stayed with me all night.

I woke up thinking everything was fine but the moment I sat up on my bed, I knew something was wrong. Mom made a quick call to my primary care physician, Dr. Amen. He takes care of all my bumps, bruises, and other disasters.

Appointment set, we made our way to the Loft Coffee House for a morning meeting with my editor. Things went downhill from there.

Sheri, my editor, said, "What's wrong Nissi? You look really tired."

"I hit my head last night, and I feel funny..."

"You know...your eyes are not sparkling like they usually do. I think you might have a concussion."

Since I did not want to admit that possibility, I said, "I'm fine. Let's keep working." So, we did - for about two minutes. Then the world started getting a little jiggly. Finally, we decided something was *really* wrong. Back into the van and on to the emergency room...

After spending two hours in the hospital and taking over twelve x-rays of my head, shoulders, chest, neck and nose, the diagnosis was clear: CONCUSSION. The doctor told us I would be fine in a few days.

But I needed to hear it from Dr. Amen. He always puts Humpty Dumpty back together again. With his welcoming young-Santa smile, he scolded me, "You know, you don't have to hurt yourself to come see me!" A careful adjustment (he's also my chiropractor), his healing words, and we are on our way.

I was determined my bruised brain would not slow me down, even though I felt like I was sitting in a boat on the ocean. Then, the doctor told me no screens for several days. My heart sank.

I know what you're thinking, Facebook and Instagram are not going anywhere. You're right!

But that's not why I was feeling so down. Before this, I was on a roll with my writing. I started getting very confident in my writing abilities. And I thought if I even stopped for a day, I would lose the ability to write well. Boy, the Lord had a lesson in that for me.

Day after day, it became harder for me to think clearly

and to do simple things like drive my wheelchair or even carry a conversation with a single person. I started stuttering and forgetting minuscule things. The best way I can describe it is like this:

There's this very amazing book called Pilgrim's Progress. In this book, there's a guy named Christian. Christian is carrying a pack on his back. This pack is quadruple the size of Christian.

Now, imagine that pack on my back. That's what it's like for me on a normal day. It is twice as hard for me to do anything a normal person can do. With a concussion, it would be me riding a bike uphill with that same pack. As a result, I was unable to write for one whole month.

I learned many things about myself during that time. I realized how much I take the abilities I **do** have for granted. I learned I hate feeling unproductive. In fact, I even started feeling a little depressed because of this. One the biggest things I learned is that I tried to rely on my own abilities and my strengths when it came to writing.

I remember sitting down to write and thinking, *Nissi, you're smart just start writing, darn it*. Not once did I ask the Lord for help. Not once!

By week four, I was so tired and frustrated, I finally sought out my Heavenly Father. You see, I might be a good writer or not, but God makes me a great writer. God gives me the ability to talk, to think for myself and to be His vessel in this world.

After expressing to my sister how frustrated I was with the concussion, I told her I had never felt so broken before. Which is kind of funny considering most people see me as broken.

And just like that, she reminded me of something, she said, "Nissi, you have a concussion. A concussion is a bruise. Bruises heal, and they become whole again. You are not broken!"

So, I choose to be whole. There's a Bible verse that I'm drawn to, it goes like this

Each time he said,
"My grace is all you need.
My power works best in weakness."
So now I am glad to boast
about my weaknesses,
so that the power of Christ
can work through me.
2 Corinthians 12:9 (NLT)

This does not mean I get to go around having a pity party. Complaining and boasting in my weakness are two completely different actions. For me, it's a choice I have to make daily.

"God never said that
the journey would be
easy, but He did say that
the arrival would be
worthwhile"
-Max Lucado-

27. ENCHANTED ROCK

Adopt the pace of nature: her secret is patience.
- Ralph Waldo Emerson-

Have you ever imagined something, and it turned out to be completely different in reality?

When I was 15 years old, I experienced my first adventure without my mom there to guide me.

Our youth group divided for the weekend. There were at least six youth leaders and twelve to fifteen girls. I don't remember what the boys did, but, for some reason, us girls decided to climb Enchanted Rock.

Enchanted Rock is a 425-foot-high dome made up of, well,

pretty much, rock. People come from all over the nation to Fredericksburg, Texas, to climb it. I assumed it was probably accessible. Why else would a group of girls decide to take me? So, I left Momma at home, jumped into a van with the girls, and headed to the dome.

I will never forget the first time I saw it. I froze, *Oh crap!!* "That's not it. Is it?" *Is there an elevator to the top of that thing?*

The weight of fear began to settle on my chest, but one glance from Bella relieved it immediately. Ever since we were little, all she has to do is give me a certain look, and I know she is going to take of care me. It's like she is saying, "I got you." Without saying a word.

The girls decided to take me as far as they could and have our Bible study wherever we landed. So, off we went. The youth leaders took turns carrying me with my chair over boulders and large rocks.

An hour into our climb, I thought we must be halfway to

the top by now. We had worked so hard! I couldn't believe we had only made it to the base of the actual rock! *Are you kidding me?*

Naturally, we were the talk of the town, so to speak - That crazy group of girls with the crazy idea to carry a girl in a wheelchair up the Rock. Many people offered to help, but my youth leaders kept saying, "No thanks. We got this!"

In my head I yelled, *PLEASE HELP!*

In between fits of laughter and utter fear that these women were going to drop me. The only part I enjoyed was being away from home for the day. But as we trudged along, I could tell they were getting tired, and truth be told, I didn't trust them. In fact, I barely knew them! Not only that, it was late January, and I was freezing! I could tell the leaders were losing momentum, and I felt drained. Not just physically drained, but emotionally drained.

As bad as I felt, I'm sure no one knew, because I was

really good at putting on a face, a mask. The thought of being vulnerable and showing the real me terrified me. Remember, this was the first time I had ever done something remotely adventurous without my entire support system - a.k.a. Mom! Although I knew these girls, they were relative strangers and I wasn't comfortable enough to reveal my true self.

Finally, three young guys (all football players) walked by us and offered to help. Once again, the girls refused their help, but I was screaming in my head, *HELP! HELP! HELP ME!*

I remember it like it was yesterday: The boys went up ahead of us and sat on a rock. It's vivid in my mind, even now. They drank water and just watched us. After they talked amongst themselves, they headed straight for us. "We decided, we are not gonna take 'no' for an answer. We are taking her to the top." True to their word, they did!

With the boys at the helm, we started moving much

quicker, as they pushed, pulled, carried, and generally lugged me up the rock. I began to relax and really take in the scenery. The beautiful pink granite that makes Enchanted Rock. This giant dome that sticks out from the middle of a huge oak and cedar forest.

Our climb became steeper as we kept going. So many times, the girls asked if they could help, but our sweet guardian angels ignored them and kept going. At one point, there was no way to stand up straight without gravity pulling them backwards. So, two guys in the front crawled on hands and knees, pulling, while the third guy pushed from behind, I kept repeating to myself, *Don't look down! Don't look down! Don't look down!*

Because we were moving a little slow, some of the girls had gone ahead, and our leaders lost track of them. We actually had to stop at some point for some of the leaders to go looking for the missing girls. We told the boys we would be fine without them, but, once again, they refused to leave us. In fact, one of them went looking with our leaders, while the other two kept a hold on me, trying to keep me warm. (I would be lying, if I didn't say I enjoyed the attention from BOYS!)

Finally, we made it to the top. I can recall the exact moment I sat in my wheelchair over the plate that said this was the highest point. I was overjoyed and couldn't believe I made it. Bella began to push me around, and I couldn't stop smiling. The JOY! The absolute joy at being at the top of that mountain made me so, so, so happy. I know I was nowhere near it, but I felt like I was on top of the world (which at that point in time my life was a huge deal). Like every teen-age girl, I was dealing with so many overwhelming things, like making friends and flirting with as many boys as I could. (So sad, but so true).

I can't recall how long we were up there, but by the time we were ready to go down, the boys were nowhere in sight. They had very strictly told us, "Come find us before you head down the hill. Do NOT try to go down without us!"

Did my leaders listen? Of course not!!

Why didn't I open my big mouth? I'm still asking myself that same question. Truth be told, we couldn't find them. Also, everybody thought it was going to be easy going down. You know, gravity!

Well, it wasn't!

GRAVITY! Gravity became our mortal enemy.

We were barely going over the big slope of the dome, when everybody started slipping. I don't know why I looked over my right shoulder. But when I did, I saw all three boys RUNNING down the dome to get to us like a bunch of freakin' superheroes. I wanted to jump for joy. They scolded our leaders when they finally reached us. "Why didn't you wait for us?".

"We couldn't find you, and we thought going downhill would be easier," someone managed to explain shakily.

The rest of the journey down is pretty much a haze to me. Except one incident that I remember: We were more than halfway down. The boys decided to take a break. When they were done, the dudes in the front lifted my chair, but the dude in the back wasn't paying attention...

So, like a wheelbarrow, I tumbled backwards. For a whole 10 seconds all I could hear was the crickets. Nobody moved. Nobody breathed.

Naturally, of course, I started laughing. And just like that, I eased the tension of our small party. The two guys in the front got mad at the guy in the back. They checked me for injuries, and we kept moving.

Enchanted Rock was just the beginning for me. That's why it's so important. Since that climb, I've done much harder things, but the moment Wendy, Jenny, Meg and Marin decided to take me up those pile of rocks, they planted a seed of adventure and a determination to do the impossible inside me. I have used the experience of going up Enchanted Rock in many circumstances in my life.

I used it as an example in my High School graduation speech.

"Have you ever climbed Enchanted Rock? I have. It was like High School for me. Nobody thought I could do it, like nobody thought I could graduate high school, but I accomplished both with the help of the people around me."

Climbing Enchanted Rock is one the few experiences I think about now and then to remind myself of who I am. Of where I've been and where I am today. I was so broken back then. It's a beautiful reminder, nothing is impossible for God! With him I can do anything. Even climb a mountain!

Be careful not to think of her
as the helpless girl in the wheelchair.
I began to understand that
when I heard she let a group of crazy
girls lug her up Enchanted Rock.

-Scott- (Pastor)

28. BATTLE PARTNER

And we know that God causes everything to work together for the good of those who love God and are called according to his purpose for them.
—Romans 8:28 NLT—

We all battle with lies and the voices in our heads telling us, *You can't succeed, give up!* And, *You're not beautiful. You'll never have true friends.* Etc. etc. etc.

By the grace of God, battling anxiety for three years taught me how to say "NO" to the lies.

Nevertheless, there are several lies I still struggle with today: *I can't do this alone*, and *Why me, Lord? Why me? Why did you allow this to happen to me? Why am I in a*

✝

wheelchair? Why do I have to suffer?

Screaming at the top of my lungs. Crying out to God. Pleading with him to take away the pain and everyday battle. *I can't do this alone. I can't be what people want me to be. I'm not strong enough. I'm not brave enough. I'm a fraud.* These are the thoughts that go through my mind over and over, non-stop. All daisies and roses, huh?

And just like that, the Lord meets me where I am. "Baby girl, who told you you're alone? I'm here when you're crying in your bed. I'm here with you when you're screaming in frustration. You were not born to do this alone. I'm right here. Rely on me!

"My sweet girl, you're only human. Humans make mistakes. But, the more you rely on me, the more you'll see you can do anything. Because when You are weak, I am strong. Let me carry you, baby girl! Let me show you what true freedom is. My love for you is so beyond the understanding of men."

I'm reminded daily of this with a calligraphy scripture on our bathroom wall. I love, love this scripture. It makes me feel invincible:

"...but they that wait upon the Lord

shall renew their strength;

they shall mount up with wings as eagles;

they shall run, and not be weary;

and they shall walk, and not faint."

(Isaiah 40:31 KJVA)

This scripture is precious to me, because this is what the Lord has been gently trying to pound into my thick skull my entire life. I believe I was born for victory. Dictionary.com explains victory beautifully: "A success or triumph over an enemy in battle or war."

If I was born for victory, that means I was born for battle as well. But the beauty of it is I don't **ever** have to battle alone. The Lord said he would never leave me and never forsake me. I believe that with all my heart. I have experienced His overwhelming love and security countless times. I imagine God walking beside me through it all.

He was there when I fell off a horse the first time. He was there when family life was a mess. He was even there when I thought no one knew what I was looking at on my computer. He was there when I ran the Tough Mudder.

He is always here when I scream out, because I can't take the pain anymore!

Struggle and pains are part of life. But, we were never meant to do it alone! Make sure you have someone - whether it be the Big Guy upstairs or a significant other, a friend. Take the time to find someone to walk beside you, to encourage you and remind you of your true potential.

P.S. There's this beautiful Christian song that I absolutely love because it reminds me that I'm not alone. Here it is:

A PARADOX OF VICTORY

"I am the Lord your God, I go before you now
I stand beside you, I'm all around you
Though you feel I'm far away,
I'm closer than your breath
I am with you, more than you know

I am the Lord your peace, no evil will conquer you
Steady now your heart and mind, come into my rest
Oh, let your faith arise, lift up your weary head
I am with you wherever you go..."

Come to Me by **Jenn Johnson**

She is so much more than most people, the personality, the commitment, the passions. She puts you first, she's got more invested than most people. She is going to invest in you. She actually cares for people.

—Ben— (Close Friend)

Excruciating grace, life, beauty: Nissi lives an excruciating life, but not what you think. When you meet her, you might pity her. Later, this will embarrass you AS you realize that what is excruciating about her life, is that it will not leave you alone.

—Scott— (Pastor)

When I often think of how Nissi does all the things she has done with her limitations, I realize I have no excuse. I coach basketball in a small casino town in the western U.S. The area is plagued with a victim mentality, but I wanted my players to hear her speak about her road trip with just her sister. When they see how much see can do, then they have no excuses.

—Ben— (Close Friend)

EPILOGUE

Oh, my gosh, I can't believe I just wrote this book!

To be honest, I wish I could have told you about all the amazing people and experiences I have enjoyed in my life, but my body, my brain, and a limited number of pages prevented that.

This journey has been exhilarating, traumatizing, healing, and eye-opening. To have the opportunity to look back and to see just how much the hand of God has been sustaining me my whole life. If there is anything I have learned, it is that nothing is ever black and white. So many layers, circumstances and people brought color and depth to my experiences.

If this doesn't make sense, just picture a paradox. A paradox doesn't make sense unless you dig deeper.

Learn to dig deeper. Don't ever limit yourself. Because, if I did, you would not be reading this book.

Nissi Salazar

ABOUT THE AUTHOR

Nissi Salazar was born in Maryland but got to Texas as fast as she could. Her love of nature and animals takes her outside every day to "walk" the neighborhood. Her love of people takes her into a life full of friends and new friends.

Although Cerebral Palsy is a constant in her life, her faith in the Lord goes beyond disability: She's dabbled in horseback riding and dog training, hiking, and her future definitely includes skydiving! Nissi lives in Bulverde, the front door of the Texas Hill Country.

There you will find her sharing her story of hope with any group, large or small.

Go to her website:

Nissisalazar.com

ABOUT THE CO-AUTHOR

Sheri Summers Hunt has been married to Hilton since 1983. Life-long Texas residents, and polar opposites, together they addressed various challenges of marriage and parenting to successfully raise two sons.

The author of acclaimed poetry and short stories, she actively works helping groups and individuals hone their writing and public speaking skills.

Her first book, THE OLDEST SIN IN THE BOOK, is a memoir-based Bible study about her journey from obesity to obedience. Available in workbook form, this study is changing perspectives about the impact of lifestyle overeating in the life of Christian women. Sheri is available to teach a 12-week course in the North San Antonio area. The teaching sessions will be available online in the fall of 2019...

Contact Sheri at:

sherisummershunt.com

A PARADOX OF VICTORY

✝

Made in the USA
Lexington, KY
29 September 2019